Secrets Of A Healer - Magic of Iridology

Secrets of a Healer

HEALER

VOL. V
MAGIC OF IRIDOLOGY

Dr. Constance Santego

Maximillian Enterprises
Kelowna, BC

Secrets Of A Healer – Magic of Iridology
Copyright © 2020 by Dr. Constance Santego.

Copy Editor & Interior Design: Constance Santego
Book Layout: ©2017 BookDesignTemplates.com
Cover Design: Jennifer Louie

Trade paperback ISBN: 978-0-9783005-4-8
Ebook ISBN 978-0-9783005-6-2
Created and published In Canada. Printed and bound in the United States of America

First Edition
Published by Maximillian Enterprises
Kelowna, BC
Canada
www.constancesantego.ca

Ordering Information:
Quantity sales. Special discounts are available on quantity purchases by corporations, associations, and others. Contact the "Special Sales Department" at the address above for details.

Dedication To
Dr. Bill Caradonna, my first Iridology Instructor

*We are only as blind as
we want to be.*

—Maya Angelou

Other Books
Constance Has Written

FICTION
The Nine Spiritual Gifts Series:
Journey of a Soul – (Vol. 1 Michael)
Language of a Soul – (Vol. 2 Gabriel)
Prophecy of a Soul – (Vol. 3 Bath Kol)
Healing of a Soul – (Vol. 4 Raphael)

NON-FICTION
The Intuitive Life, The Gift of Prophecy, Third Edition
Fairy Tales, Dreams and Reality... Where Are You On Your Path?
Second Edition
Your Persona... The Mask You Wear
Angelic Lifestyle, A Vibrant Lifestyle
Angelic Lifestyle 42-Day Energy Cleanse
Archangel Michael's Soul Retrieval Guide

SECRETS OF A HEALER, SERIES:
Magic of Aromatherapy (Vol. I)
Magic of Reflexology (Vol. II)
Magic of The Gifts (Vol. III)
Magic of Muscle Testing (Vol. IV)
Magic of Iridology (Vol. V)
Magic of Massage (Vol. VI)
Magic of Hypnotherapy (Vol. VII)
Magic of Reiki (Vol. VIII)
Magic of Advanced Aromatherapy (Vol. IX)
Magic of Esthetics (Vol. X)

FOR CHILDREN

I am big tonight. I don't need the light!

Contents

Preface

The Miracle of Iridology

I remember my first day studying Iridology. It made no sense at all to me. I looked at hundreds of eyes; all I noticed was the color. It was like learning braille. A whole new language. The story that your eyes tell.

The study of the iris is fascinating. I can tell by looking into your eyes the constitutional state you inherit. I can tell what system in your body is your weakest link, and in time if you do not look after yourself, it will be the one that causes your demise.

By the end of that weekend's introductory course, I knew I could tell what was wrong with you, but what in the world do I do now? How do I fix you?

It has been twenty-two years since that weekend, and since then, I have learned many ways how to fix you.

To me, that is the best gift any person could ever have. The gift of premonition—the state of your health before anything terrible happens. The bonus of knowing which system of your body you need to look after so that you remain healthy!

I have found this true in all the years I have been practicing the healing arts. So, what if I know how to fix you, the point is the real power is in learning how to heal yourself.

P.S. No matter where life brings me, I write these books always to have access to this amazing knowledge. The manuals are also part of my legacy for my children and grandchildren.

Enjoy, Dr. Santego

Note to Reader

Iridology is not to replace modern medicine. Iridology is a tool, a map of our body. It has no power to heal you on its own. It can only tell you what system in your body you need to keep healthy.

Your Doctor still plays a vital role in your health care. For example, if I break my leg, I will need a Doctor and all the nurses and staff that work in the Hospital to help me heal.

I follow Eastern Medicine's belief "That **we play** a significant role in our health care." What we put into our bodies, how hard we work our bodies, the stress level we allow into our everyday life, and the amount of positive or negative energy we attract around us all play a role in our well-being.

Shift happens...Create magic!

Learning Outcome

When you have completed this book and studied the concepts and techniques, you will be able to see markers in your eyes that can tell you which system may have trouble with if you abuse it.

- Know And Understand What Iridology Is
- Identify Structural Signs In The Iris
- Be Able To Chart What You Found
- Know Your Overall Physical Resiliency
- Know Your Resiliency Subtypes, Modifiers, and Iris Constitution
- Ideas For What You Can Do With Your Findings
- Know Your Basic Emotional Iridology

PART ONE

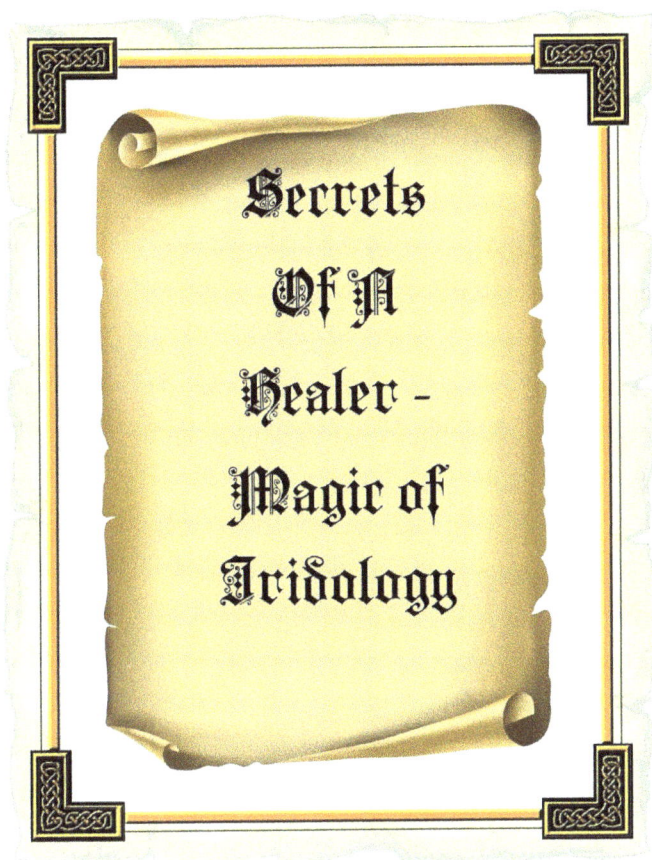

Secrets Of A Healer - Magic of Iridology

What is Iridology?

Wikipedia version:

Iridology (also known as iridodiagnosis or iridiagnosis) is an alternative medicine technique whose proponents claim that patterns, colors, and other characteristics of the iris can be examined to determine information about a patient's systemic health.

Practitioners match their observations to iris charts, dividing the iris into zones corresponding to specific human body parts. Iridologists see the eyes as "windows" into the body's state of health.

- Iridology studies markings mapped out in the left and right iris.
- Sclerology studies markings in the eye's white part (Sclera).

Bernard Jensen's version

Iridology is a method whereby the doctor or health practitioner can tell, from markings or signs in the iris, the reflex condition of various organs and systems of the body. These markings represent a detailed picture of the body's integrity, constitutional strength, congestion or toxic accumulations, and inherent strengths and weaknesses.

Dr. Constance Santego's version

Iridology tells me what you were born with, Reflexology tells me what you have been up to, and Massage tells me where you hold all your emotions and issues.

Iridology is a critical piece of the puzzle.

Brief History

I was taught that Iridology was discovered by accident, literally.

When only a boy of ten years, a Hungarian, Dr. Ignatz von Peczely, was playing with an owl in his hometown of Egervar, near Budapest, unfortunately, he happened to break one of its legs.

I could imagine his horror as the bird stared back at him. Then, as history has it, he noticed the appearance of a dark stripe in the lower region of the bird's iris. Eventually, this black streak became a tiny black spot, around which were white lines and shading.

At the age of 36, he became interested in medicine and studied first in Budapest in 1862. In 1864 he went on to Vienna. In 1866 he started practicing in Budapest and published his first book on the iris, "Discovery in the Realm of Nature and Art of Healing" This work was made known in Germany by August Zoeppritz. Dr. Emil Schlegel of Tuebingen published a book on the results of von Peczely's work.

The incident with the owl impacted the mind of the future doctor. Working in the hospital's surgical wards, he started to observe the eyes of all his patients. When they came in from an accident and before and after their operation, years later, he found that this darkened area in the iris corresponded to the location of the owl's broken leg. In this manner, he was enabled to construct the first chart of the iris.

Living many miles apart and not knowing each other, Nils Liljequist, a Swedish homeopath, wrote similar books simultaneously, even writing word for word in many instances. Nils writings were translated into two volumes called "Diagnosis from the Eye." Nils brought his work of iridology to America.

Dr. Henry Edward Lane, a native of Austria, came to this country and taught iridology to Dr. Henry Lindlahr from Chicago. Doctor Lane wrote the first iridology book published in this country, entitled "iridology, the Diagnosis from the Eye." This book was copyrighted and is in the Congressional Library in Washington. The sixth edition was published in 1904.

Doctor Lindlahr, as Doctor Lane's student, gave iridology serious study and applied it in his work in natural therapeutics. He wrote a valuable reference book entitled "Iris Diagnosis," which is Volume VI of his library on natural cures.

Other scientists also have used and contributed to this science.

- Peter Johannes Thiel of Germany is considered one of the great iridologists of the day.
- Dr. J. Kritzer has written a splendid textbook called "Iris Diagnosis and Guide in Treatment".
- Dr. Marko J. Petinak and Dr. F. W. Collins have contributed charts.
- Dr. R. M. McLain of Oakland, California, has taught this science for many years.

The person who brought iridology into the twentieth century was Bernard Jensen, and carrying on his work was his daughter Ellen Tart-Jensen.

Two Belief Systems

Question? Do the various features of the iris represent a permanent aspect of an individual's health, <u>or</u> will the iris shift and change throughout their life in response to their behavior?

The different schools of iridology seem to answer this question differently and in shades of grey. For the purposes of this course, we can break the schools into two general groups:

Belief A:

The iris is a "snapshot" of a single point in a person's life and can change due to various stresses and Hering's Law of Cure. Acquired problems and weaknesses appear when the fibers split apart, showing the layers below.

The iris is constructed in five layers, as seen in the cross-section of the iris.

To illustrate the process of a lesion formation, reflecting the condition of a weaker organ, let us take the example of a person coming down with a cold. When a person ends up with a cold, it reflects an irritated lung mucus condition. In the iris, a portion of the lung area, at approximately 2:30 in the left iris, will show swollen tissue fiber that is raised and whitest in color in a blue iris. Likewise, a brown iris will show a lighter brown color in the region. These fibers will appear to rise off the surface of the iris, reflecting an acute condition in the lung.

Acute means a condition in its active stage of inflammation; coughing, sneezing, with a running nose, or spitting up mucus. Acute conditions, anywhere in the body, will appear as raised tissue whiter or lighter in color.

At this stage, the outcome is dependent on what the person does. So, we need to step back and look at what the body is trying to do. People who believe in natural therapies don't believe in the post-Pasteurian theory that you "catch a cold."

You do not just catch a cold for one reason or another. Probably there was a low level of vital energy in the lungs, along with an accumulation of morbid mucus. The mucus with low vital energy is a breeding ground for the virus, thus producing a catarrh. The word catarrh is derived from the Greek - "to flow." Part of the process of a cold is to encourage the morbid mucus to flow out of the body, taking toxic materials with it. What do you do if you use a pharmaceutical that relieves the symptoms of a cold? You dry up the mucous membranes, crystallizing the mucus so it cannot flow. Yes, you relieve the symptoms of the cold, but do you overcome the problem? The answer, of course, is "no." All that you do is drive the toxins deeper into the tissue. This gives us a symptom-free situation but brings us to the second level of inflammation.

Belief B:

Iris markings **<u>do not</u>** change over a person's life.

They are just a blueprint of the person's composition (general makeup).

These markings would show us what <u>could</u> happen to a person if they <u>abuse</u> their body.

Since 1992, I have been studying Iridology and my own eyes. I have had many changes in that time, and with all the pictures I have taken so far, there has been no change to my eyes.

Remember, it takes three similar markings to even mean that there <u>may</u> be a severe issue/trait.

This book is based on this belief system, "B," until science proves this differently.

What You Can & Cannot Identify

What Iridology Can Identify, from Jensen & Bodeen, Visions of Health, 1992.

hat Iridology CAN identify...

- The primary nutritional needs of the body.
- The inherent strength or weakness of organs, glands, and tissues.
- Constitutional strength or weakness
- Which organs are in the greatest need of repair and rebuilding?
- The relative amount of toxic settlement in the organs, glands, and tissues.
- Where inflammation is located in the body.
- The stage of tissue inflammation and activity.
- Under activity or sluggishness of the bowel
- Spastic and ballooned conditions of the bowel.
- The need for acidophilus in the bowel
- Prolepses of the transverse colon.
- A nervous condition or inflammation of the bowel.
- High-risk tissue areas in the body that may be progressing toward a disease.
- Pressure on the heart
- The circulation level in various organs.
- Nerve force and nerve depletion.
- Hyperactivity or hypoactivity of organs, glands, and tissues.
- The influence of one organ on another or the contribution of an organ to a condition elsewhere in the body
- Lymphatic-system congestion.
- Poor assimilation of nutrients.

- Depletion of minerals in an organ, gland, or tissue.
- The relative ability of an organ, gland, or tissue to hold nutrients.
- The results of physical or mental fatigue or stress on the body.
- The need for rest to build up immunity.
- Tissues areas contributing to suppressed or buried symptoms
- High or low sex drive.
- A genetic pattern of inherent weakness and their influence on other organs, glands, and tissues.
- The effects of iatrogenic conditions.
- The preclinical stages of diabetes, cardiovascular conditions, and many other diseases
- Miasms
- The recuperative ability and health level of the body.
- The buildup of toxic material before the manifestation of a disease.
- Genetic weaknesses affecting the nerves, blood supply, and mineralization of bone.
- The genetic influence on any symptoms present.
- Healing signs indicating an increase of strength in an organ, gland, or tissue.
- The potential for varicose veins in the legs.
- Positive and negative nutritional needs of the body.
- A probable allergy to wheat
- Sources of infection.
- The acidity of the body and catarrh development.
- Suppression of catarrh
- The condition of tissues in any one part of the body, or in all the parts of the body at one time.
- The climate and altitude that is best for the patient.
- The potential for senility.
- The effects of a polluted environment
- Adrenal exhaustion

- Resistance to disease.
- The relationship or unity of symptoms with conditions in the organs, glands, and tissues.
- The difference between a healing crisis and a disease crisis.
- The accuracy of Hering's Law of Cure
- Whether a particular program or therapy is working.
- The quality of nerve force (nerve energy) in the body.
- The body's response to treatment.
- The whole, or overall, the health level of the body.

What Iridology CANNOT identify...

- Blood pressure levels (normal or abnormal), blood sugar level, and other specific diagnostic findings and laboratory test results
- Which specific medications or drugs an individual is using or has used in the past.
- What surgical operations a person has had
- Specifically, what foods a person does and does not eat.
- How much uric acid is in the body?
- The time and cause of an injury to the body.
- Whether a snake bite is poisonous and if the snake venom has entered the bloodstream.
- The correlation between tissue inflammation levels and specific diseases or symptoms or disease.
- Diseases by name.
- Whether a subject is male or female.
- Whether asbestos settlements or silicosis exist in the body.
- If your hair is falling out and why.
- The number of organs with which a person was born

- The presence of a yeast infection, such as Candida albicans.
- Which tooth is causing problems?
- The presence of lead, cadmium, aluminum, or any other metallic elements in the tissues.
- If a woman is on birth control pills.
- If a woman is pregnant.
- Whether an operation is necessary
- Whether a tumor is present and what size it is.
- Whether Hemorrhage exists in the body or where it is located
- The difference between drug side-effect symptoms and the symptoms of actual diseases.
- Whether irregular menstrual periods are caused by the thyroid
- The presence of multiple sclerosis, Parkinson's disease, or bubonic plague.
- Whether healing signs indicate a rising of the general health level.
- The presence of syphilis, gonorrhea, or another sexually transmitted disease.
- Orientation toward homosexuality.
- The presence of AIDS
- The presence of gallstones or kidney stones.
- Whether a cardiac artery is blocked.

Who Can Be Tested?

To be very accurate, anyone over the age of twenty-five. Eyes can change up to the approximate age of twenty-two. After that, you are left with your life's physical and emotional constitution.

Babies are born with blue eyes, and then within hours, the eye color starts to change. If a guardian knew what to look for in the child's eyes, they could alter that child's diet and lifestyle to bring homeostasis—balance.

Most of us were not raised with this belief, and if not already, we will soon be dealing with our health issues.

If you can answer yes to any of these questions, it may disqualify you from your true and factual iridology results.

- Have you ever had an eye injury? Yes ___ No ___
- Have you ever had eye surgery or laser treatment? Yes ___ No ___

An eye injury or surgery will most likely have left a scar of some kind or some tissue may have been removed or altered, causing the markings you find to be false.

- Do you wear a contact lens? Yes ___ No ___
  Color _____

If you remove the contact lens and have not had an injury or eye surgery, you should be able to see any markings you might have.

Reading The Eyes

Tools Needed

To look into your own eyes, purchase a lighted magnifying mirror. There used to be a company called ContacScope that sold a handheld self-examine magnifying glass. If you can find one of those, grab it.

In the past, I have taken pictures with a camera and recently with my cell phone. The best way is to purchase an excellent but very expensive Iridology Camera.

To look into other people's eyes, all you will need to purchase is a lighted magnifying glass. There are many different powers that you can buy. The two that you will need will be a 5x power for blue eyes and a 10x power for dark brown eyes. You can purchase these magnifying glasses at any pharmacy, Eye Dr. Office, or online.

To Examine:

Sit on a chair with your legs on one side of the client's chair. *You may want a breath freshener (certs or tic tac) first.*

When you are ready to read the client's eyes, have one hand lightly touching the client's head or shoulder before you come in with the magnifying glass. Make sure you always hold the magnifying glass firmly in your hand.

*Note: a client can only keep their eyes open without blinking for a short period of time with the light so bright. So, he/she may need to take an occasional moment break now and again.

As you go through this information, look at as many different eyes as possible. Practice looking at friends and family member's eyes or anyone who will let you take a peek. Even look at people's eyes in magazines.

Do not tell anybody what condition you think they have. ONLY A DOCTOR IS ALLOWED TO DO THAT!!!

We are not allowed to diagnose!

If need be, tell them what marking you are looking for. Later, when you are confident, you may tell them about their personality and what body systems they need to focus on.

Anatomy of The Eye

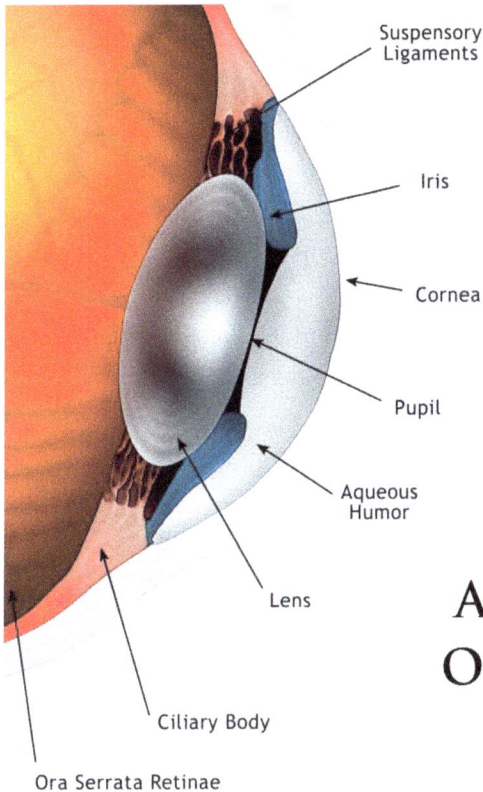

ANATOMY OF THE EYE

Labels: Suspensory Ligaments, Iris, Cornea, Pupil, Aqueous Humor, Lens, Ciliary Body, Ora Serrata Retinae

Iris

A colored, muscular ring that controls the amount of light entering the eye. It lies underneath the cornea, in front of the lens, and within the sclera.

Cornea

The transparent layer of tissue that covers the eyeball.

Pupil

The aperture within the iris allows light to enter the eye. Behind the eye sits a translucent lens which focuses the incoming light Lens can become cloudy, a condition known as cataracts.

Lens

This allows the focusing of light on the back of the inside of the eyeball (retinal surface), lies behind both the pupil and the iris, and is suspended with its own set of ligaments.

Sclera

It is the white of the eye, often containing visible blood vessels. It is covered by a translucent layer called the cornea.

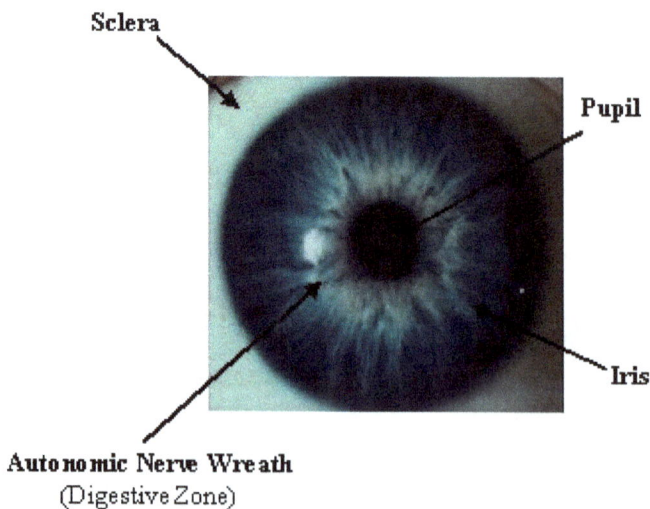

Sclera

Pupil

Iris

Autonomic Nerve Wreath
(Digestive Zone)

Systems of the Body

CARDIOVASCULAR / CIRCULATORY SYSTEM

Anatomy

> Heart, arteries, and veins

Function

> Transport oxygen and nutrients to the cells, remove metabolic wastes from the cells and tissues and carry hormones from one part of the body to the other.

Suggestions to help you with this system:

> Nutrition, minerals, water, Aromatherapy, Herbs, and Exercise. Massage, Reflexology and Shiatsu.

ENDOCRINE SYSTEM

Anatomy

> Pituitary, pineal, hypothalamus, thyroid, parathyroid, thymus, adrenal, pancreas, ovaries, and testes.

Function

> Regulate and integrate the body's metabolic activities, and maintain homeostasis.

Suggestions to help you with this system:

> Aromatherapy, Herbs, Meditation, Reiki, Shiatsu, Reflexology, and Energy Techniques.

DIGESTIVE SYSTEM

Anatomy

> Mouth, salivary gland, tongue, esophagus, stomach, gall bladder, liver, pancreas, large intestine (colon), small intestine, and rectum.

Function

> To process food & eliminate wastes from the body.

Suggestions to help you with this system:

> Food (what is being put into the mouth), the digestive system needs fiber to move the food through and lots of water. The rest of the body needs the proper nutrients to survive—exercise (movement will help to process the food). Aromatherapy, Herbs, and Relaxation a stressed system cannot process the food properly.

INTEGUMENT / SKIN

Anatomy

> The largest organ of the body

Function

> It protects against invading pathogens, regulates the body temperature via perspiration and shivering, provides a waterproof covering for the body, and receives information about the outside world.

Suggestions to help you with this system:

> Since it is one of our eliminating organs, keeping it clean is very important to our detoxifying process. Herbs, Spa, Massage, and Aromatherapy techniques can be used here.

IMMUNE SYSTEM

Anatomy

> Tonsils, sinuses, appendix, spleen

Function

> To defend the body against attack from infectious organisms and other harmful invaders (aka pathogens)

Suggestions to help you with this system:

> European Lymph Drainage Massage, Aromatherapy, and Herbs, Keep the bodies vibration balanced

LYMPHATIC SYSTEM

Anatomy

> Lymph nodes, axillary's lymph nodes, cisterna chyli, inguinal lymph nodes, mammary plexus, thoracic duct

Function

> Production of lymphocytes throughout the body, drainage of intestinal fluid back into general circulation.

Suggestions to help you with this system:

> Nutrition, minerals, water, and exercise (especially bouncing and walking) are important. European Lymph Drainage Massage, Aromatherapy, Herbs, and Reflexology are beneficial.

MUSCULAR SYSTEM

Anatomy

> There are 640 named muscles in the body and thousands of unnamed ones.

Function

> To permit movement

Suggestions to help you with this system:

> Nutrition, minerals, water, and exercise are essential. Relaxation, Aromatherapy, Herbs, Reiki, Reflexology, Muscle testing, Yoga, Tai chi, Qui Gong, Shiatsu, and Massage.

NEUROLOGICAL SYSTEM

Anatomy

> Brain, hypothalamus, spinal column, and nerves

Function

> It is to relay information in the form of nerve impulses throughout the body, thereby controlling its functions.

Suggestions to help you with this system:

> Aromatherapy, Herbs, Meditation, Yoga, Tai chi, Qui gong, deep breathing, relaxation, energy techniques, Reiki, Shiatsu, Reflexology, Massage (Chair, Hot Stone, Swedish or ELD), and Spa techniques.

REPRODUCTION SYSTEM

Anatomy

> Women- uterus, ovaries, fallopian tubes, vagina.

> Men- prostrate, testicles, scrotum, seminal vessel.

Function

> Females- produce ovum, produce offspring. Males- produce sperm and fertilize the ovum.

Suggestions to help you with this system:

> Nutrition, minerals, water, and exercise are essential. Relaxation, Aromatherapy, Herbs, Reiki, meditation, Reflexology, muscle testing, yoga, Tai chi, Qui gong, Shiatsu, and massage.

RESPIRATORY SYSTEM

Anatomy

> Nose, trachea, bronchi, bronchioles, lung, diaphragm

Function

> Oxygen - carbon dioxide exchange via inspiration and expiration, maintaining proper acid-base balance in the blood, and speech production.

Suggestions to help you with this system:

> Aromatherapy, Herbs, Meditation, Yoga, Tai chi, Qui gong, deep breathing, exercise, and Swedish massage.

SKELETAL SYSTEM

Anatomy

There are 206 skeletal bones

Function

Protection, locomotion, production of red and white blood cells by the bone marrow, and storage of minerals such as calcium and phosphorous.

Suggestions to help you with this system:

Nutrition, minerals, exercise, and weights are essential. In addition, aromatherapy and Herbs are beneficial.

URINARY SYSTEM

Anatomy

Kidneys, ureters, bladder, urethra

Function

Separate certain waste products from the blood helps maintain the blood at a constant level of composition.

Suggestions to help you with this system:

Nutrition, minerals, water, and exercise are essential. Relaxation, Aromatherapy, Herbs, Reiki, and Reflexology.

SPECIAL SENSES

Function

Sight, hearing, taste, smell, and touch.

Suggestions to help you with this system:

Energy techniques, Muscle Testing, Aromatherapy, Herbs, Reiki, Reflexology, Shiatsu, Meditation, and Massage.

PARASITES

Anatomy

It is an organism that obtains its food and shelter by living on or in another organism.

Function

Parasites only come when the body goes into an acid state which tells the universe the body is dying and it needs to be decomposed.

Suggestions to help you with this system:

Keep the body health on all levels, and do a parasite cleanse at least once a year.

Hering's Law of Cure

Three principles:

1. All cure comes from above downward.
2. All cure comes from within, out.
3. All symptoms leave the body in the reversal of the order they enter it.

These three statements can be understood on many levels, and as you work with the principles, new applications of it will appear.

1. All cure comes from above downward. If you do not want to be healthy, you will not be. You have to think, feel and desire to be healthy. Many people, some of whom you will no doubt run into, want to be sick. It is a crutch for them to lean on. They receive the attention they otherwise would not. Something for them to feel sorry about a healthy attitude is an essential ingredient in a healthy body.

2. All cure comes from within, out. The most vital organs and the most vital parts of an organ will be cured first. Your body will spend more energy on strengthening the health of the liver than spending energy on arthritis in the knee.

3. All symptoms leave the body in the reversal of the order they enter it. Let's say, as in our preceding discussion, a person went through a degeneration process such as a cold, flu, bronchitis/pneumonia, hay fever, or asthma—a degenerative lung issue. If this person came into the natural healing clinic and were put on a good

natural diet and given the proper herbs, vitamins, and other supplements, they would feel much better after a while. The typical response from someone like this after a few months is:

"You know I feel so much better, you would not believe ... I can sleep a whole night through now. Before, I could only get a short rest sitting in a chair because when I laid down, I felt like I was drowning in the mucus from my lungs. Thanks, you know you saved my life. I'll do anything you say from now on. I'm deeply indebted to you."

These are warning words to a well-versed practitioner. The patient's vital energies have been raised enough to rid their body of many toxins they have acquired to create their devitalized state in the first place. This person is about to have a healing crisis.

Healing Crisis

A healing crisis is when the body has gained enough vital energy to eliminate some accumulated toxins in the devitalized tissue. The same person, who a week earlier was praising the ground you walked on, might phone back and call you all kinds of names because they are now sicker than a dog." In this case study, they would come down with a bad case of asthma just when they thought they were cured. In a healing crisis, you relive the old symptom set, and it often becomes even worse than before, but usually for very short periods, until the accumulated toxins are released. The release of these old toxins is often associated with eliminating drugs that might have been taken during the period of the original disease symptom.

A healing crisis is always preceded by a period of high vital energy and is followed by a period of high vital energy associated with a feeling of release. This whole process of revitalization of the tissue in question can go on until each of the previous symptom sets experienced has gone through a reversal in the order in which they entered the body, with a healing crisis at each stage until the tissue is completely healed.

The past opinion of healers was that we had to go through all the healing stages. We have found in our practice this is not necessarily true. A well-trained practitioner can often avoid the need for a major healing crisis, though it will crop up from time to time. For example, if a person goes on long cleanses, trying to vitalize the body quickly, they will have many healing crises. But if they take a slower route, cleanse a little, build a little, cleanse a little, build a little, we can often avoid major healing crises.

Some herbal formulas are perfect for this. They may be designed with both slow-cleansing and building properties. This brings the person back to a fully vitalized body by a slower, often more comfortable, path. Changing one health level to another is like changing gears in a car. Sometimes you might "grind the gears" a little, but you can switch the gears smoothly with care.

One of the most common questions is, "How can you tell the difference between a healing crisis and a disease crisis?" Of course, a healing crisis has a good level of vitality on both sides. But you know, to distinguish them apart is little more than an academic exercise. As Doctor Kellogg said:

"You give me any crisis, and I can heal that person of all ailments." When we go into a crisis, whether up the road toward vitality or down the path to a degenerative-type situation, our body is in a state of "health alert," meaning it can call upon particular energies to heal. Let us not forget that fact while reviewing the disease process we discussed at the beginning of the lesson. These were confirmed cases of the body trying to rid itself of toxins and morbid waste.

If you follow the simplest of the laws of nature in a crisis, including plenty of rest, very simple food (maybe just liquid), the right vitamins and minerals, and sometimes herbs to assist in the elimination process, you can rid the body of the problem and most often, the organisms associated with it. You have to act before they have too much of a stranglehold.

Eye Color Determination

Most babies are born with blue or grey eyes and will start to change color within hours. It takes about a year for melanocytes to finish their work. The color change does slow down some after the first six months of life, but there can be plenty of change left at that point, right up to the age of Twenty-two.

When we talk about eye color, we are talking about the appearance of the iris, the muscular ring around the pupil that controls how much light enters the eye. As a result, eye color varies depending on the lighting conditions, especially for lighter-colored eyes.

Other factors influence your eye color, such as pigment and heredity.

Pigment Formation:

In humans, the pigmentation of the iris varies from light brown to black, depending on the concentration of melanin in the iris.

Over time, if melanocytes only secrete a little melanin, you will have blue eyes. If they secrete more, your eyes will look green or hazel. When melanocytes secrete a lot of melanin, eyes look brown (the most common eye color), and in some cases, they may appear Black.

Heredity:

Your genetic constitution is a visual expression of your eye color. The choice of eye color is determined by an allele found on a specific locus position on your chromosome.

Depending on what eye color your parents have, it will determine what color you will most likely have.

Homozygotic - Brown eye color - the *B* allele confers brown eye color

Heterozygotic - Both brown and blue eye color - recessive *b* allele gives rise to blue eye color

Heterochromia - Complete heterochromia is when a person has two different colored eyes. Heterochromia of the eye is caused by variations in the concentration and distribution of melanin, the pigment that gives color to the skin, hair, and eyes.

In grade 10 Biology class, you may have learned about two parents having a baby, what color of eyes will the children have?

Examples of eye color

B B = True Brown eyes (iris is a dark brown color)

B b= Hybrid Brown eyes (iris is various colors of brown)

b b = True Blue eyes (iris is various colors of blue; digestive wreath can be yellow to dark brown)

Figure #1

If both parents have True Brown eyes – B B

- Their children have a *100%* chance of having true brown eyes

Parent A (Mom) True Brown Eyes—B B

	Child B B	Child B B
Parent B (Dad) True Brown Eyes—B B	Child B B	Child B B

Parents A and B have True Blue eyes.

- Their children have a *100%* chance of having True blue eyes.

Fact: *If you have both parents with true blue eyes and you have hybrid brown eyes, then you were either adopted or your mom had a different partner.*

Figure #2

If both parents have Hybrid Brown eyes – B b,

- Their children have a 25% chance of having true brown eyes
- 50% chance of having hybrid eyes
- And a 25% chance of having true blue eyes.

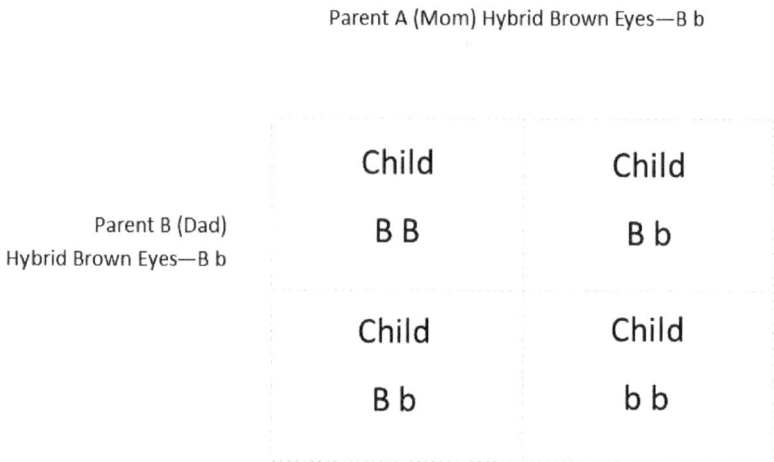

Parent A (Mom) Hybrid Brown Eyes—B b

Child B B	Child B b
Child B b	Child b b

Parent B (Dad) Hybrid Brown Eyes—B b

Figure #3

Parent A has Hybrid Brown eyes, and parent B has True Brown eyes.

- Their children have a 50% chance of having True brown
- And a 50% chance of having Hybrid eyes

Parent A (Mom) Hybrid Brown Eyes—B b

	Child B B	Child B b
Parent B (Dad) True Brown Eyes—B B	Child B B	Child B b

Map Of The Eyes

FOR CHARTING

Location Zones

To read the eyes, we first must understand the graphing procedure. Just as the Earth is graphed into degrees of longitude and latitude, Continents and then into Countries and so forth for us to locate a specific location, so are the eyes.

Pupillary & Ciliary Zones:

Both the right and left eyes are divided into Pupillary & Ciliary Zones

The Pupillary and Ciliary zones divide the iris into four equal parts.

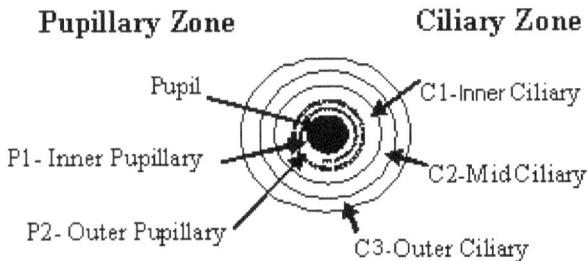

The pupillary zone is from the pupil to the inside of the Digestive or Autonomic Nerve Wreath.

The pupillary zone is further divided into two equal parts:

P1- Inner pupillary

P2- Outer pupillary

The Ciliary Zones are from the outside of the Autonomic or Digestive Wreath to the Sclera (white of the eye).

The Ciliary Zone is divided into three equal parts:

C1- Inner Ciliary

C2- Mid Ciliary

C3- Outer Ciliary

Function Zones

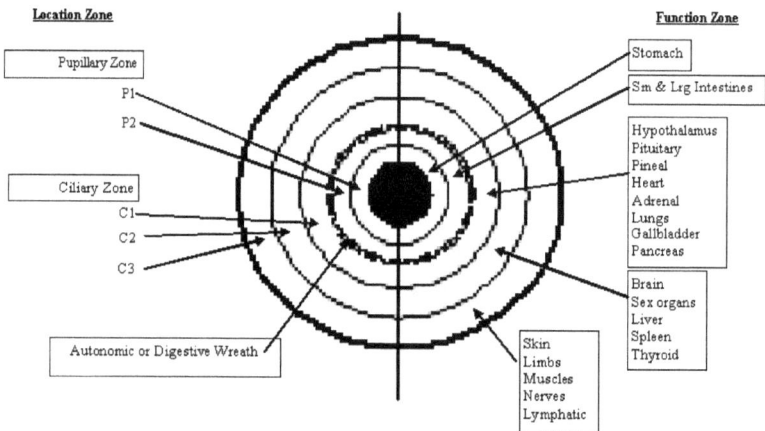

Location Zone — Function Zone

Pupillary Zone
P1
P2

Ciliary Zone
C1
C2
C3

Autonomic or Digestive Wreath

Stomach
Sm & Lrg Intestines
Hypothalamus
Pituitary
Pineal
Heart
Adrenal
Lungs
Gallbladder
Pancreas
Brain
Sex organs
Liver
Spleen
Thyroid
Skin
Limbs
Muscles
Nerves
Lymphatic

The iridology markings that you will focus on with the body's different systems are in these zones of the iris.

Cardiovascular / Circulatory System

Anatomy

Heart, arteries, and veins

Function

Transport oxygen and nutrients to the cells, remove
metabolic wastes from the cells and tissues and carry
hormones from one part of the body to the other.

Suggestion

Nutrition, minerals, water, Aromatherapy, Herbs, and
Exercise. Massage, Reflexology and Shiatsu.

Digestive System

Anatomy

Mouth, salivary gland, tongue, esophagus, stomach, gall
bladder, liver, pancreas, large intestine (colon), small
intestine, and rectum.

Function

To process food & eliminate wastes from the body.
Refer back to page 19 to analyze the digestive system.

Suggestions

For food (what is being put into the mouth), the
digestive system needs fiber to move the food through
and lots of water. The rest of the body needs the proper
nutrients to survive—exercise (movement will help to
process the food). Aromatherapy, Herbs, and
Relaxation a stressed system can not process the food
properly.

Endocrine System

Anatomy

> Pituitary, pineal, hypothalamus, thyroid, parathyroid, thymus, adrenal, pancreas, ovaries, and testes.

Function

> Regulate and integrate the body's metabolic activities, and maintain homeostasis.

Suggestion

> Aromatherapy, Herbs, Meditation, Reiki, Shiatsu, Reflexology, and Energy Techniques.

Integument / Skin

Anatomy

> The largest organ of the body

Function

> It protects against invading pathogens, regulates body temperature via perspiration and shivering, provides a waterproof covering for the body, and receives information about the outside world.

Suggestion

> Since it is one of our eliminating organs, keeping it clean is crucial to detoxifying it. Herbs, Spa, Massage, and Aromatherapy techniques can be used here.

Immune System

Anatomy

Tonsils, sinuses, appendix, spleen

Function

To defend the body against attack from infectious
organisms and other harmful invaders (aka pathogens)

Suggestion

European Lymph Drainage Massage, Aromatherapy,
and Herbs balance the body's vibration.

Lymphatic System

Anatomy

Lymph nodes, axillary's lymph nodes, cisterna chyli,
inguinal lymph nodes, mammary plexus, thoracic duct

Function

Production of lymphocytes throughout the body,
drainage of intestinal fluid back into general circulation.

Suggestion

Nutrition, minerals, water, and exercise (especially
bouncing and walking) are essential. European Lymph
Drainage Massage, Aromatherapy, Herbs, and
Reflexology are beneficial.

Muscular System

Anatomy

> There are 640 named muscles in the body and thousands of unnamed ones.

Function

> To permit movement

Suggestion

> Nutrition, minerals, water, and exercise are essential. Relaxation, Aromatherapy, Herbs, Reiki, Reflexology, Muscle testing, Yoga, Tai chi, Qui Gong, Shiatsu and Massage.

Neurological System

Anatomy

> Brain, hypothalamus, spinal column, and nerves

Function

> It is to relay information in the form of nerve impulses throughout the body, thereby controlling its functions.

Suggestion

> Aromatherapy, Herbs, Meditation, Yoga, Tai chi, Qui gong, deep breathing, relaxation, energy techniques, Reiki, Shiatsu, Reflexology, Massage (Chair, Hot Stone, Swedish or ELD), and Spa techniques.

Reproduction System

Anatomy

Women- uterus, ovaries, fallopian tubes, vagina.

Men- prostrate, testicles, scrotum, seminal vessel.

Function

Female- produce ovum, produce offspring.

Male- produces sperm and fertilizes the ovum.

Suggestion

Nutrition, minerals, water, and exercise are essential. Relaxation, Aromatherapy, Herbs, Reiki, meditation, Reflexology, muscle testing, yoga, Tai chi, Qui gong, Shiatsu, and massage.

Respiratory System

Anatomy

Nose, trachea, bronchi, bronchioles, lung, diaphragm

Function

Oxygen - carbon dioxide exchange via inspiration and expiration, maintaining proper acid-base balance in the blood, and speech production.

Suggestion

Aromatherapy, Herbs, Meditation, Yoga, Tai chi, Qui gong, deep breathing, exercise, and Swedish Massage.

Senses

Function

Sight, hearing, taste, smell, and touch.

Suggestion

Energy techniques, Muscle Testing, Aromatherapy, Herbs, Reiki, Reflexology, Shiatsu, Meditation, and Massage.

Skeletal System

Anatomy

There are 206 skeletal bones

Function

Protection, locomotion, red and white blood cell production by the bone marrow, and storage of minerals such as calcium and phosphorous.

Suggestion

Nutrition, minerals, exercise, and weights are essential. Aromatherapy and Herbs are beneficial.

Urinary System

Anatomy

Kidneys, ureters, bladder, urethra

Function

Separating certain waste products from the blood helps maintain the blood at a constant level of composition.

Suggestion

Nutrition, minerals, water, and exercise are essential. Relaxation, Aromatherapy, Herbs, Reiki, Reflexology.

Extra: **Parasites**

Anatomy

An organism obtains its food and shelter by living on or in another organism.

Function

Parasites only come when the body goes into an acid state, which tells the universe that the body is dying and needs to be decomposed.

Suggestion

Keep the body health on all levels, and do a parasite cleanse at least once a year.

Degrees of a clock:

Imagine the iris as a clock for both the right and left eyes.

The top is 12:00 o'clock and reading clockwise.

I start at 12:00 and work around the left eye and then proceed to do the same to the right eye. I take notice of any color changes and structural markings within each zone in that time section. Finally, I draw a mock-up eye and place my findings on it.

NOTE: Remember the Iridology Map (Simplified Research Chart) is as if you are looking at the person's eyes. When you are looking at your own, the map is reversed.

Iridology
Simplified Research Chart

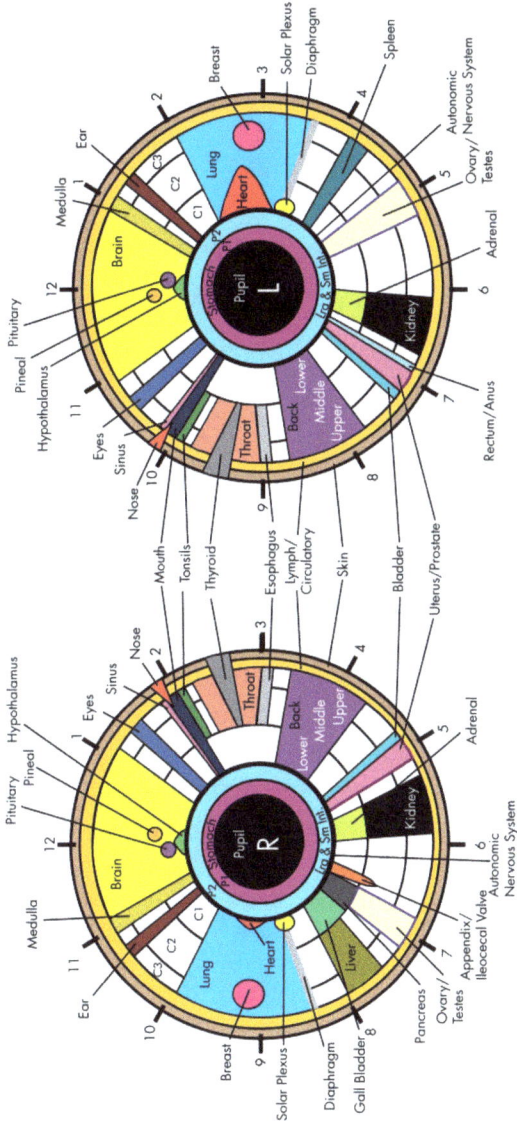

Structural Signs
The Three Main Ones

#1 Physical Integrity

There are many structural signs to look for when you are an Iridologist. In this book, I will introduce you to the easiest ones to notice with significant meaning.

For physical integrity, it takes three to five similar structural signs before you can say that a system of the body is weakened and needs care. Each eye marking counts as one point, but the question is, what system of the body gets the point? There are eleven body systems, plus your senses:

- Digestive
- Muscular
- Skeletal
- Nervous – Central and Peripheral
- Lymphatic
- Circulatory – Blood
- Immune
- Urinary
- Genital
- Reproductive
- Respiratory
- Senses; sight, hearing, taste, smell, and touch

If you look at the map of the eyes, each of these body systems is in both the right and left eye. Each structural sign you find counts as one point. Color also counts as a point.

Note: *You can also do Iridology for Emotional Integrity.*

Total Rating of ALL the Physical Integrity: As you review the list, markdown 1 – 10. 10 is good, and at the end, add the point amounts and divide by the # of physical integrity you listed.

This will tell you your overall resiliency constitution (how fast you bounce back from an illness).

> Example: If you caught a cold
>
> > 8 - 10 is a couple of days
> >
> > 4 – 7   is about a week
> >
> > 1 - 3   is a couple of weeks

RESILIENCY

The iris is composed of two sphincter muscles formed by many fibers that resemble the spokes of a wheel and together act like the adjustable aperture of a camera.

This background identifier indicates the measure of the ability to work hard with reduced physical stress, decreased frequency of illness, increased recuperative abilities, and greater longevity potential. It also indicates the abuse capacity of the body.

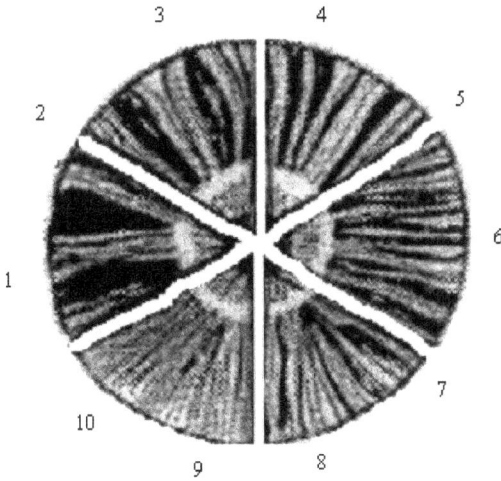

The closer these **fibers** are, the better the parts' resiliency (10), genetic strength, or constitution.

An analogy that is used:

An oak desk: Oak has a very tight grain and can take much abuse without showing it. It can easily withstand a blow and continue to function. In contrast, a pine desk has a softer consistency and a greater tendency to show damage. Drop something sharp or hard on a pine desk, which may show the results forever.

Resiliency Scale

1-2 = Pinewood   or Burlap material

3-4 = Fir wood   or Muslin material

5-6 = Oakwood   or Cotton material

7-8 = Maple wood   or Rayon material

9-10= Iron Wood   or Silk material

People with a strong resiliency/constitution (tight-fibered irises) can "get away" with more than people with loose-fibered irises.

You have heard of the big guy being able to eat two hot dogs, three hamburgers, French fries, drink lots of beer, and keeps on going. But, haven't you wondered how they can still be healthy? They have strong resiliency/constitutions! Where other people become sick with the slightest change from a perfect diet. These people usually have weaker resiliency. A common term for this quality is tissue reserve.

The greater the individual's overall tissue reserves, the greater the resources they can call upon in times of stress or poor nutrition. Often these strong, resilient individuals abuse themselves terribly when they are young because they can take it, and around age 45-50, they go to the doctor saying, "I've never been sick a day in my life, but lately I just feel run down" or "Why do I have arthritis? I've been athletic and healthy my whole life. "The abuse catches up sooner or later, even if you have a strong resiliency.

People with weak resiliency often teach young people to walk a narrower health path and enjoy life to the fullest because they have not abused their life's vital energies.

Notice the thickness and layers of iris fibers. 1 being mildly resilient (burlap/Pine) 10 being extremely resilient (silk/ironwood). **10 is the healthiest, with the most vitality.**

Integrity Rating Scale 1-10:

1	6	10

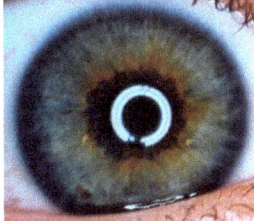
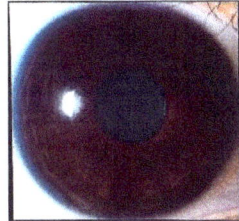

The more fibers, closer together, and the more layers
an iris has, the more resilient that person is!

#2 Lacunas

Lacuna (plural lacunae) is Latin for "pit" or "hole," relating to lacune or "lake." Lacuna is the word the Europeans use for lesions. As stated, lacunae are exactly like lesions with various levels of inflammation: acute, sub-acute, chronic, and degenerate. AKA flower

Appearance: Distinctly rounded deficiency of tissue. It resembles a flower petal.

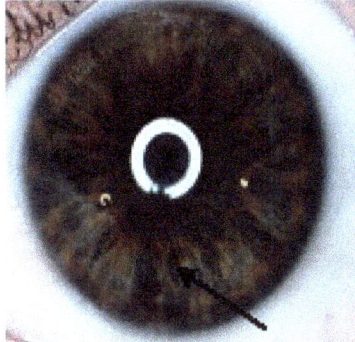

Physical Constitution Meaning:

Indicates decreased vitality or functional capacity of organs or systems.

Leaf Lacuna

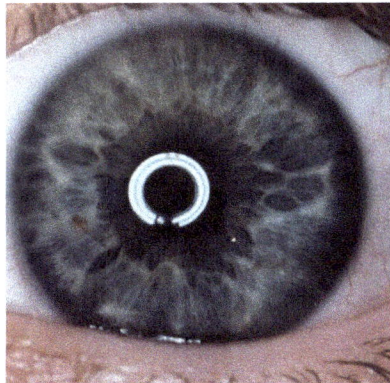

NOTE: There are many different shapes of Lacunas (open, closed, pear, lance, torpedo, step, shingle, honeycomb, crypt, and asparagus). When charting, each Lacuna counts as one point in its specific body system.

Open Lacuna

Appearance:

Borders of lacuna do not come together.

Meaning:

It can be an area of expression of symptoms as a "safety valve" for vitality to maintain balance.

Pear Lacuna

Appearance:

Pear shape

Meaning:

This lacuna is the precursor of the much-feared asparagus lacuna and is supposed to indicate a strong tendency toward cancer (Again, no running to the washroom mirror to look for problems. These are "research" indications and do not always indicate severe problems).

Lance Lacuna

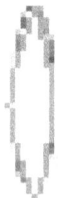

Appearance:

Tight/skinny leaf lacuna

Meaning:

Also a forerunner of the asparagus lacuna, the lance lacuna indicates a predisposition towards possible degenerative problems such as cancer.

Torpedo Lacuna

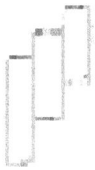

Appearance:

Tear drop

Meaning:

Large torpedo lacunae represent genetic weakness, according to some European researchers.

We had seen these lacunae when there was no indication of "normal" genetic weakness.

Smaller versions of this shape are considered to represent tumors or possibly cysts in the indicated area.

Step Lacuna

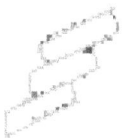

Appearance:

Vertical rectangular shapes joined together

Meaning:

This shape indicates that there is a weakness in the pancreas.

Shingle Lacuna

Appearance:

Slanted rectangular shapes joined together.

Meaning:

Shingle lacunas are basically the same as step lacunae but are "tipped over' and also represent pancreas weakness.

Honeycomb Lacuna

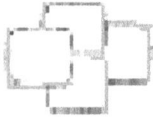

Appearance:

Joined squares resemble a bee hive honeycomb.

Meaning:

Europeans feel this represents an endocrine imbalance. It also often means a general mineral deficiency.

Crypt / Rhomboid Lacuna

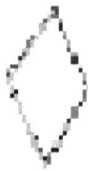

Appearance:

Diamond or rhomboid-shaped openings are located directly inside and outside the bowel wreath. It is also the classic shape of the heart lesion known as the heart diamond.

Meaning:

Reflects decreased nutrient exchange, pocketing, or defects in bowel tissue. It is typically seen in the glandular zone. This may mean Diabetes mellitus, hypoglycemia, etc.

Asparagus Lacuna

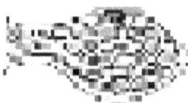

Appearance:

Look like the tip of an asparagus.

Meaning:

Some Europeans feel that this lacuna represents a 99% probability of cancer.

#3 Flecks

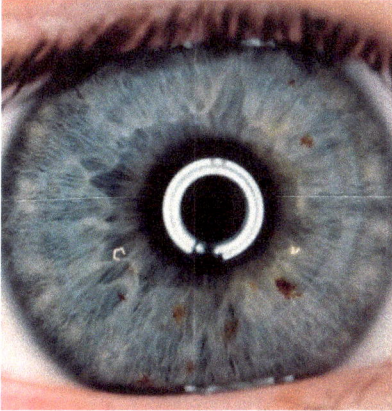

Spots of color are randomly distributed about the iris, also referred to as harmless iris freckles, medically called iris ephelis.

NOTE: Each fleck on the map counts as a point toward the specific location and system it resides in.

Topostable Pigments (fleck) - Individual

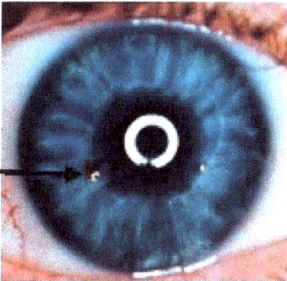

Appearance: Color fleck, singular pigments that are significant due to appearance or location.

Meaning: Indicators of potential stress or reactivity in the region.

Topolabile Pigments (flecks) - Scattered

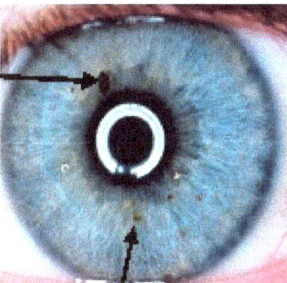

Appearance: Color flecks, general pigment pattern scattered through the iris.

Meaning: Coloration indicates system susceptibility.

NOTE: Each Fleck counts as one point in the specific body system.

Resiliency Subtypes

Every individual line, shape, and color means something. Each practitioner has a reason for why they are looking for specific markings. I use iridology to find the primary catalyst. The system in the body will create an imbalance, causing disharmony.

These markings, Connective tissue, Polyglandular tissue, and Neurogenic tissue all play a vital part in telling the whole 'Physical Constitution' story.

- A person with a neurogenic iris has more resilience than the other two. They would bounce back faster if they were to get sick.

#1 Physical Constitution:

Appearance

Observe layers or depth of iris tissue and density of fibers. The greater the amount of fibers, density, and layers, the higher the resiliency.

Meaning:

The more layers and the closer the fibers are, the more resiliency. If the person does not abuse themselves, they have more resiliency = healthier life.

Resiliency Subtype #1 - Connective Tissue

CONNECTIVE TISSUE TYPE

Rating: 1- 4 maximum

Meaning: Predisposition to connective tissue weakness reflected in organ ptosis (esp. abdominal), varicosities, and spinal anomalies and subluxations

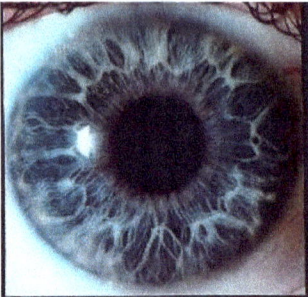

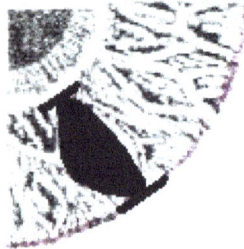

Appearance: The loose weave of stroma throughout the iris.

NOTE: In this picture, the lacuna's that <u>touch</u> the outer edge (connect) ciliary zones *always touch C1-C3 (inner thru outer)*.

Resiliency Subtype #2 - Polyglandular

POLYGLANDULAR TISSUE TYPE

Rating: minimum 4 – 7 maximum

Meaning: Tendency for deficient output of secretory glands, usually digestive (pancreas & gallbladder) and hormonal (adrenal, pituitary, and thyroid).

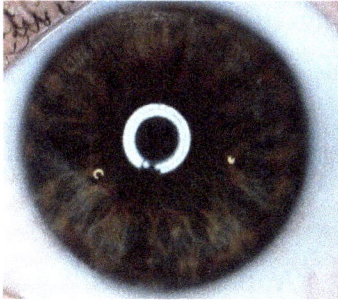

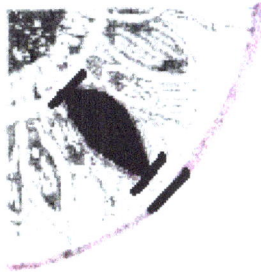

Appearance: Daisy petal' pattern of lacunae around the collaret wreath.

NOTE: Notice the Lacunas that <u>do not touch</u> the outer edge. Notice, some of the lacunas are only in the ciliary zones 1-2 (inner thru mid), not zone 3. *They are all sizes and can be anywhere*

Resiliency Subtype #3 - Neurogenic

NEUROGENIC TISSUE TYPE

Rating: minimum 7 – 10 maximum

Meaning: Increased resilient nature.

Often diligent, hardworking, industrious, without appearing stressed.

Differentiation between ROBUST and DEFICIENT variations is important.

The risk for nervous system exhaustion and headaches from vascular spasms.

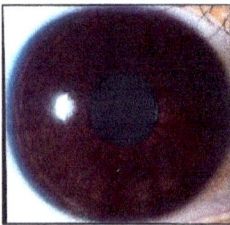

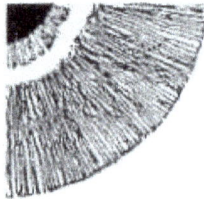

Appearance: A combination of thin, stretched, and/or delicate fibers is frequently seen with a small pupil.

Robust - Many layers and great density

Deficient - Few layers and less density

NOTE: There are NO Lacunas

Resiliency Modifiers

These next two markings will tell me:

- Contraction Furrows -about the person's ability to handle stress
- Digestive Zone - their digestion, how they take in energy

Contraction Furrows

Contraction Furrows are also known as; Stress rings and nerve or cramp rings.

Appearance: Contraction Furrows are circular rings, usually in the mid and outer ciliary zones. It can be seen with Neurogenic subtypes and less frequently with Polyglandular types, and infrequently with Connective Tissue types.

Rating 1= many and very deep and thick, 9 = hardly any and very, very faint.

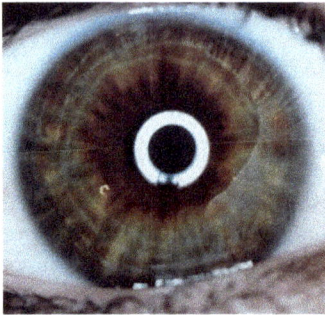

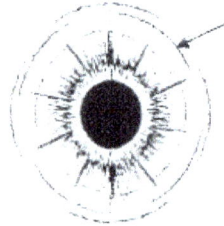

Decreases proper breathing and increases neuromuscular tension and spinal subluxations.

Decreases calcium availability, esp. in Brown eyes.

Muscular cramping increases (watch chest, abdominal, & upper back areas) and TMJ (temporal mandible joint disorder).

Indicator for attraction to stress.

Many projects are going on at once, not enough hours in the day, never a dull moment, and life is in the fast lane.

Like a wound-up spring.

If pushed to the extreme, nervous breakdown behavior is exhibited.

Deep tissue work, aerobic exercises, and deep breathing are indicated.

Digestive Zone

Digestive Zone also is known as; Autonomic Nerve Wreath, Digestive Wreath, and Bowel Wreath.

This Digestive Wreath divides the two zones.

Please take notice of the textures of the fibers. They are very different between the Pupillary 2 and Ciliary 1 Zones.

Rating:

- Balanced is a 10
- Anything else varies between 1- 9

Appearance: Balanced Wreath = 10   Not Balanced Wreath -too big or too small = 1- 9

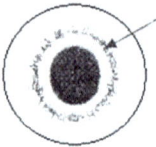

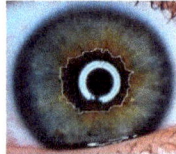

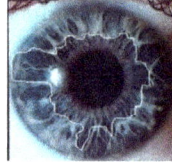

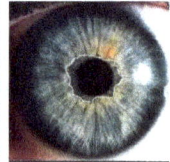

How your bowels are working will usually determine your state of health.

PLACEMENT

Divides Pupillary 2 and Ciliary 1 Zones

Notice if the wreath placement is:

A- Balanced (wreath is ¼ of the iris) what we want
Meaning: Balanced

B- Constricted (less than ¼ of the iris)

Meaning: Constipation, hard or no stool

C- Relaxed/atonic (more than ¼ of the iris)

Meaning: Constipation, loose stool, diarrhea

Rating Balanced is a 10

Constricted and Relaxed are 1-9 depending on severity.

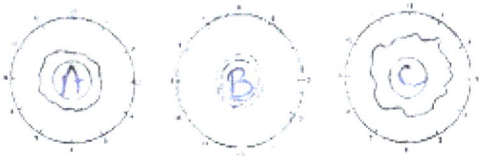

| 10 | 2 | 5 |

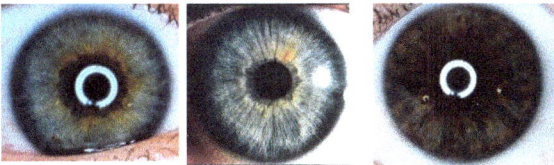

QUALITY

Quality – (wreath itself)

Notice if the wreath quality is (thick, raised, or ropy) (thin, wispy, or delicate) (absent wreath).

> A- Thick, raised, or ropy wreath
>   Meaning: Overactive
> B- Thin, wispy, or delicate wreath
>   Meaning: Sensitive, irritable
> C- Absent wreath
>   Meaning: Under active
> D- Balanced
>   Meaning: What we want, balanced

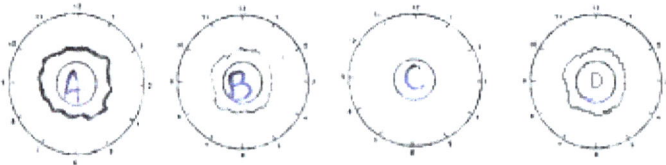

Rating Balanced is a 10

Thick, raised or ropy, Thin, wispy or delicate, absent wreath are 1-9 depending on severity.

2	4	1	10

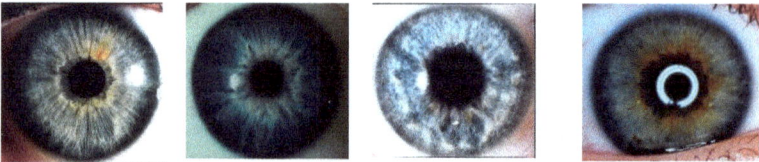

Thick	Thin/Wispy	None	Perfect

SHAPE

LOOSE OR CONSTRICTED BOWELS

The further out the digestive zone is, the looser the stool – diarrhea rating 1, tighter to the pupil equals constricted bowels – constipation rating also 1.

Notice if the wreath shape is (jagged or star-shaped) (double wreath) (intermittent wreath)

> A- Jagged or Star shaped wreath
>   Meaning: Loose stools under pressure
> B- Double Wreath
>   Meaning: Extra sensitive and irritable
> C- Intermittent wreath (start/stop)
>   Meaning: Irregular pattern of over and under active
> D- Balanced
>   Meaning: What we want, balanced

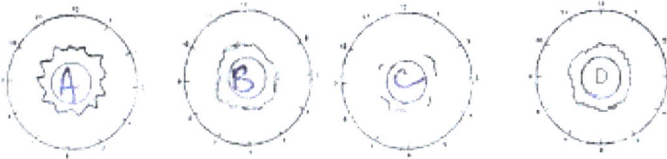

| 3 | 6 | 5 | 10 |

Rating Balanced is a 10

Jagged or Star shaped wreaths, Double Wreath, Intermittent wreath (start/stop) are 1-9, depending on severity.

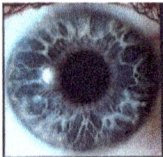

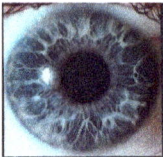

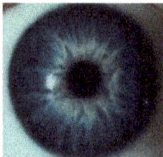

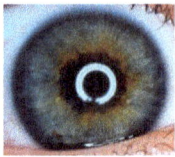

Crazy shape   also double   starts & stops   Perfect

Iris Constitution/Genotypes

EYE COLOR RATING –
1) LYMPHATIC (BLUE EYES)

Rating: 1 - 4 maximum

Blue eyes are due to a lack of melanin pigment.

All three pictures shown are considered blue eyes:

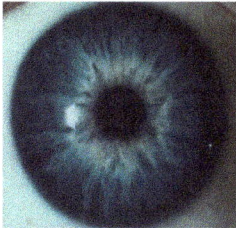

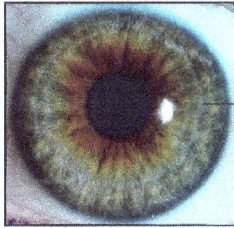

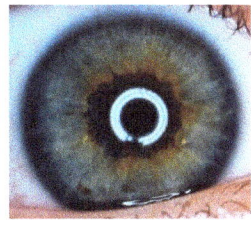

Lymphatic (Blue eyes)

- The tendency for excess mucous production and discharges with a focus on the upper respiratory, lower respiratory, alimentary, and urogenital tracts.
- Overactive immune system and allergies, over acidity, and lymphatic congestion are often present.
- Dairy is particularly mucous forming.
- Increasing the position to eczematic.

2) HYBRID / MIXED BILIARY (BROWN EYES)

You will never see any blue in them.

Rating: minimum 4 - 7 maximum

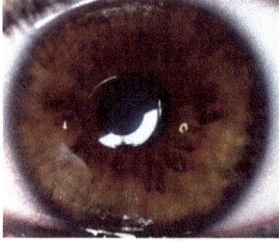

Hybrid (Brown eyes)

Light brown pigment overlaying visible white/yellowish fibers.

• Focus on the liver, gall bladder, and associated digestive disturbances.

• Often aggravated by dietary errors.

3) HEMATOGENIC (TRUE BROWN EYES)

Rating: minimum 7 – 10 maximum

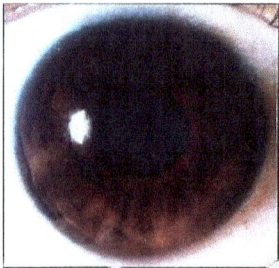

Hematogenic (True Brown eyes)

Original nationalities of; Asians, First Nations, East Indians, etc.

Brown pigment 'carpet' obscuring iris and fibers.

• A tendency to disorders of blood composition.
• The liver and gastrointestinal areas are also a focus.
• Observe for endocrine disturbances.

It is essential to know the variables of a person's health that will impact their speed of healing or what is contributing to their dis-ease:

- How fast a person can heal.
- If a food causes them issues (allergies and such).
- How they handle stress.
- How sensitive or intuitive they are to sense their own body.

Over the years, iridology has helped me understand my client's body and how to empower them.

This next section gives me more detailed information on their constitution, but honestly, I use this knowledge to tell the story of their basic personality.

- Personality traits

The easiest Markings to see are:

- Over Acidity/Febrile
- Hydrogenoid/Uric Acid
- Scurf Rim
- Ferrum Chromatose
- Cholesterol Ring/Lipemic Diathesis

Over Acid

Lymphatic eyes only!

Rating 1 - 4

Appearance:
Blue eye with whitish fibers.

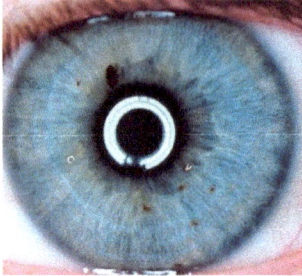

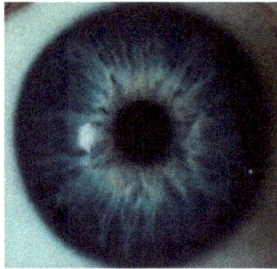

- Kidneys require extra support.
- Allergies - Acidic - arthritic nature aggravated by over-acid foods: Meat - esp. red, coffee, chocolate, white flour, white sugar, dairy, alcohol, over acid citrus, and tomato/eggplant family.

Febrile

Lymphatic eyes only!

Rating 1 - 4

Appearance:
Extremely white fiber appearance.

Kriege calls this the "steel grey" eye (white fibers have a greenish or yellowish tinge).

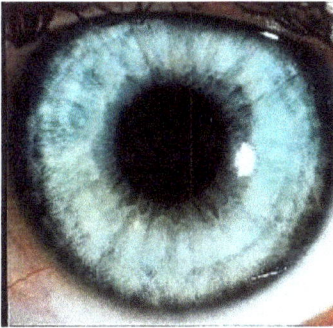

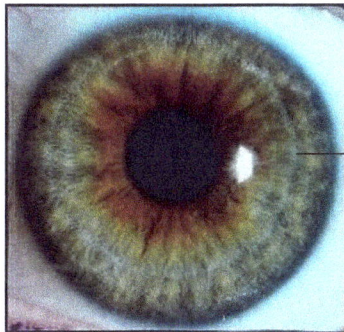

- Feverish nature, especially as a child.
- Suppression increases acidic, arthritic risk, with extra stress on the kidneys.

Hydrogenoid / Lymphatic Rosary (Cotton balls)

Lymphatic eyes only!

Rating 1-4

Appearance:
Tophi (tiny cotton balls) connective tissue bundles - in the outer ciliary 3 zone.

It can range in appearance from distinct to poorly defined and from white to discolored.

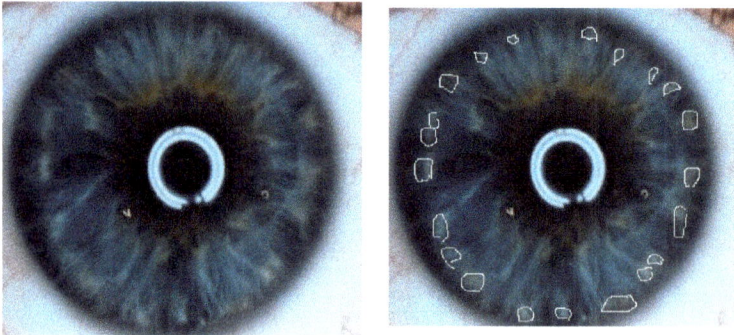

- Extra risk for lymphatic congestion and immune system overactivity.

Uric Acid

Lymphatic eyes only!

Rating 1-4

Appearance:
Thick tophi (big cotton balls) plaques in the ciliary 2 zone.

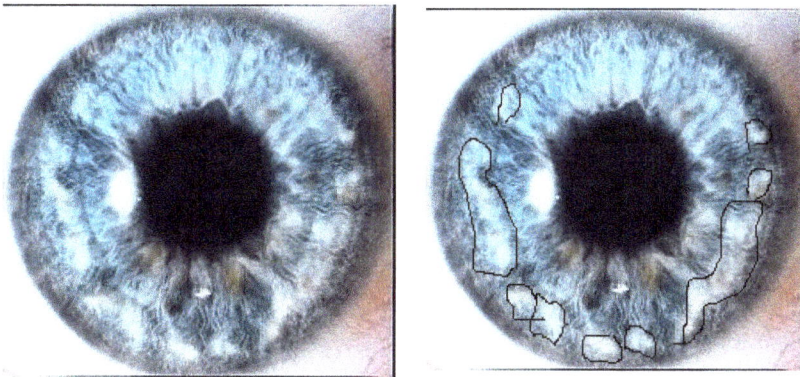

- Excess uric acid re-absorption. Irritation to kidneys and increased incidence of gout, gouty arthritis, kidney stones (esp. calcium oxalate), and cardiac irritation.

Scurf Rim

Rating 1-7

Appearance:
Darker distinct ring in the outer ciliary 3 zone.

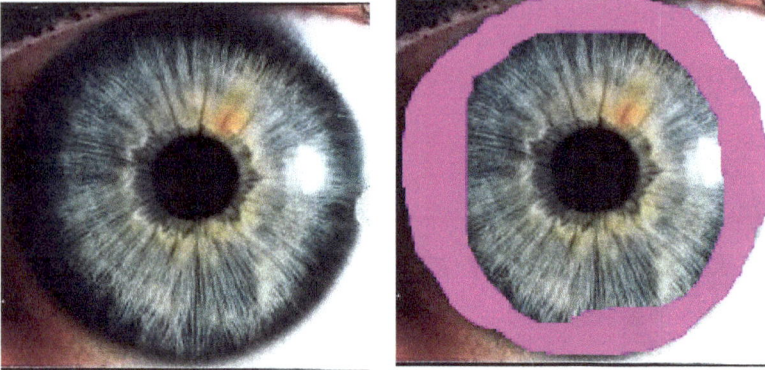

- Increased mucus production. Decreased skin elimination stresses the kidneys.

Ferrum Chromatose (Tiger striping)

Not in Lymphatic or Hematogenic eyes!

Rating 4-7

Appearance:
Bands of small dark "snuff tobacco "pigments accumulate on the surface of the iris.

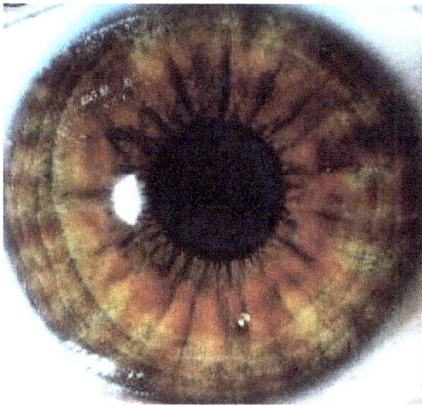

• Extra emphasis on the liver. It can indicate "wear and tear." Pay extra attention to areas where pigment has settled, especially if accompanied by other signs.

Lipemic Diathesis / Cholesterol Ring

Rating 1 - 10

Cholesterol Ring / Lipemic Diathesis / Corneal Arcus

Appearance:
White or yellowish color ring, usually in C3. Fat deposition in the outer cornea (ciliary 3) obscures the view of iris fibers. Not a true iris sign comes with age and cholesterol levels.

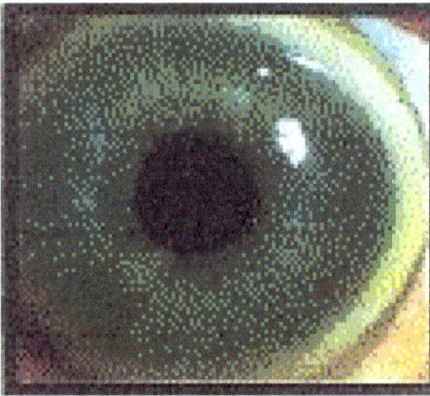

• Increased errors in fat metabolism when seen in the ages of the '40s, '50s, and '60s. Risk of arteriosclerosis and cardiovascular problems.
• Also, the liver, pancreas, and thyroid insufficiencies. Normal aging signs when seen in later life.

Note: *It is the only marking I have witnessed change in an adult.*

Miscellaneous Structural Signs

Physical Integrity #1 - Iris Pigmentation (color):

After determining the background pigmentation of the iris constitution (Brown, Hybrid of Blue), there are other localizes and specific pigments.

In most cases, color indicates reduced organ functional capacities or increased susceptibility to stress. In addition, the color could determine the inflammation, toxicity, or acidity level in the person's body.

If blue or brown eyes have these colors in the iris, the system of the body that could be affected be:

Color	Meaning
Straw Yellow -	Kidney
Orange -	Pancreas and Liver
Fluorescent Orange -	Gallbladder, Pancreas, and Liver
Brown - (light, medium, dark, reddish)	Liver
Black/Tar -	Pre-cancerous and Liver

Physical Integrity #2 - Radial Solaris

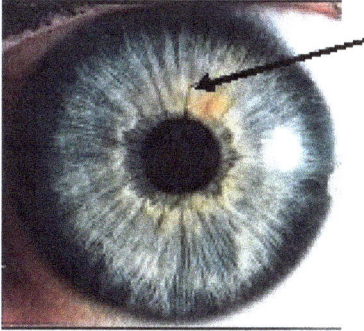

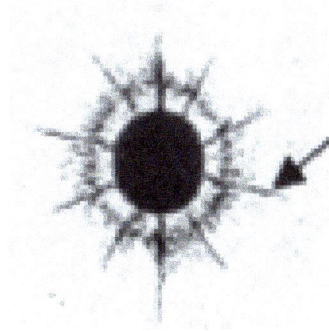

Appearance:

Notice the spoke-like lines that radiate out from the pupil.

Meaning:

- Each line indicates a low level of seepage from the intestinal tract into the area represented on the chart.
- Thus, producing a low level of septicemia (septic blood) and inflammation.
- This area may be high in parasite activity.

Physical Integrity #3 - Radial Furrows

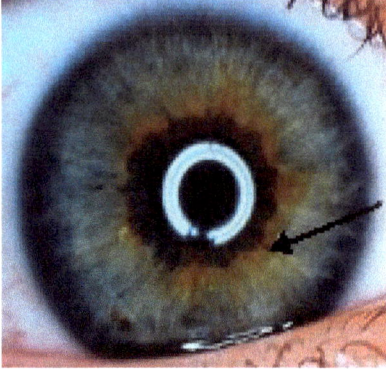

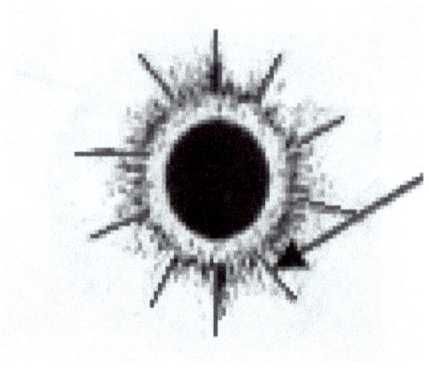

Appearance:

NOTE: Notice the spoke-like lines that radiate from the ciliary 1 zone / autonomic nerve wreath, not from the pupil as in the previous picture.

Meaning:

- This indicates increased toxic material in the adjacent and surrounding tissue.

Physical Integrity #4 - Transferrals

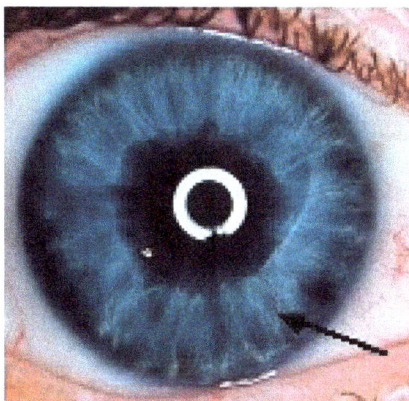

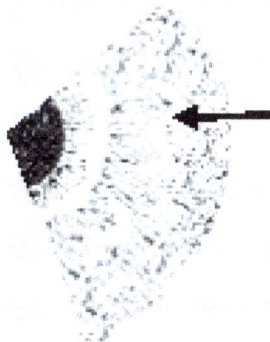

Appearance:

Reflexive fibers that transverse the normal direction
(squiggly sideways line)

Meaning:

- Irritation inflammation or pre-cancerous genetic
  indicators

Physical Integrity #5 - Pupil Tonus

<u>Pupillary Change</u>

The specific purpose of the pupil is to allow light into the eye. The muscles in the iris structure which accomplish this action are the sphincter pupillae and dilator pupillae. Both muscles are under the control of the autonomic nervous system, namely the sympathetic arid parasympathetic. When there is pressure on the spinal cord's nerve root, such as spinal subluxation, a reflex action occurs, and the pupil flattens across from the area serviced by the particular nerve supply.

> For example. If there is nerve root pressure in the upper cervical spine, say C-1, the pupil will flatten on the frontal portion (12 o'clock).

In this way, the pupil can tell the iridologist where there is nerve interference in the entire body and which areas it affects. According to research, the pupil will eventually return to its corrected shape by correcting the nerve root pressure in the body.

The "pupil tonus" is a term used in iridology that refers to the observation of pupil flattening and deformation. To the iridologist, pupil tonus can be another means of clarifying and cross-checking for iris signs in the analysis. The observance of the pupil tonus is noted as a "sectoral flatness" to various sides of the pupil, such as frontal, temporal, nasal, and ventral. The occurrence of pupil deformation signifies the deviation of the circular shape of the pupil and indicates a severe disturbance. The pupil tonus chart developed by Harri Wolf is valuable for observing pupil tonus arid deformation.

Check to see what size the pupils are to start with (E.g., dilated). This will guide you if the iris is stretched or relaxed. Relaxed markings may look wider; the next time you look, if the pupils are stretched, you may think that healing occurred when nothing has happened.

Appearance: Flattening or Elliptical shape of the pupil

 Elliptical- shape indicates a stroke history in the family. Observe for other cardiovascular risks in the patient.

 Flattening- indicates spinal subluxation tendencies specific to certain locations.

It can have more than one flattening on each eye and can have both Flattening and Elliptical.

Elliptical Pupils	Meaning

Direction of pupil

Right eye/Left eye

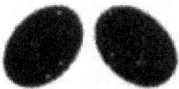 1) Weakness and motor disturbances in the lower extremities with possible paralysis. Pains due to muscle spasms extending from the buttocks down.

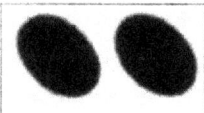 2) Right-sided paralysis. Genito-urinary disturbances.

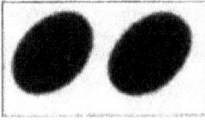

3) Left-sided paralysis. Sexual disturbances. Lack of strength and energy in the legs.

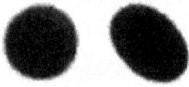

4) Nervous asthma. The left bronchus is more seriously disturbed.

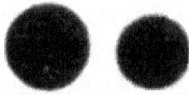

5) A background of hereditary syphilitic damage (if there is no history of diphtheria or meningitis)

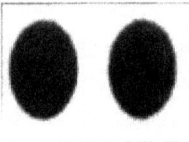

6) Impending cerebral hemorrhage or clotting (coma or paralysis may follow)

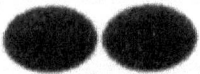

7) Glandular disturbance with influence upon the heart and respiration (check the thyroid). Depression. Motor disturbances.

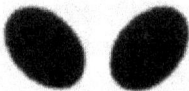

8) Anxiety states, neuroses, weeping, spells, and muscle spasm. Tendency to cerebral hemorrhage and paralysis.

Flattening Pupils   Meaning

Direction of pupil

Right eye/Left eye

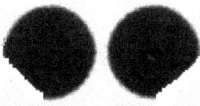

1) Weakness in arm and shoulder movement. Irritation and possible subluxation T1-4, T6 & 7 vertebrae. Hepatic insufficiency.

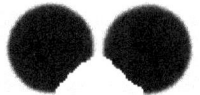

2) Irritation to the Sacral/Lumbar region of the spine and its associated neural pathways. Genital-urinary disturbances. Arthritic and Rheumatic signs.

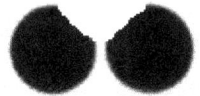

3) Irritation & possible subluxation to the cervical vertebra. Visual problems. Digestive & Hepatic insufficiencies.

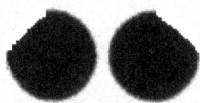

4) Hearing difficulties. This may be due to dilation of the cerebral vessels or tumors in the cerebellum.

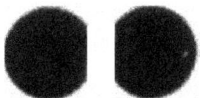

5) Restriction to breathing (the heart may be affected). Possible subluxation C1-5 vertebra.

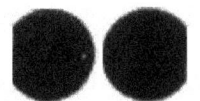

6) Nervous breathing. Possible impending circulatory collapse.

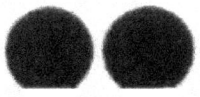

7) Weakness in the pelvis & lower extremities. Poor elimination abilities. Possible persistent headaches.

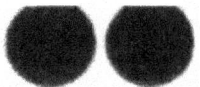

8) Tendencies to depression, fatigue, paranoia, melancholy, and guilt feelings. Possible subluxation of Cl vertebra.

Physical Integrity #6 - Central Heterochromia

Appearance: Orange color (color varies) digestive zone

"Opposite" pigment around the pupil, generally in the digestive or nutrient transport and assimilation zone

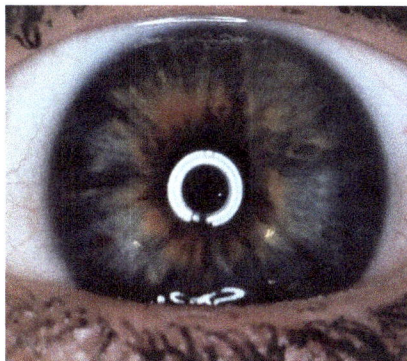

Meaning: Increased challenges or focus on digestive and intestinal function.

Physical Integrity #7 - Sectoral Heterochromia

Appearance: Orange color (color varies) on iris C1-C3

Opposite" pigment in a section of iris.

Varies in size and extension to the iris edge

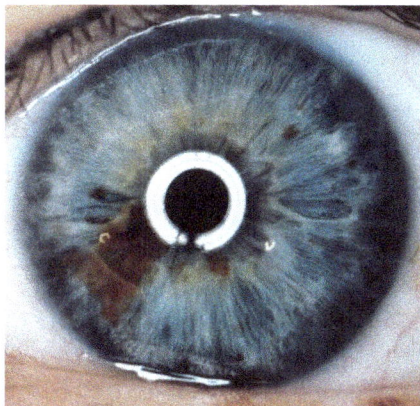

Meaning: Genetic marker; may be significant depending on color and location.

Physical Integrity #8 - Arthritic Netting

Appearance: Whitish web around the outer ciliary zone 3, usually only seen in blue eyes.

Meaning: Increased Arthritic tendency

Physical Integrity #9 - Defects

Appearance: Small openings or holes in the ciliary zone of the iris tissue.

Meaning: Lowered activity or vitality in a specific area.

Physical Integrity #10- Perifocal Lightening

Appearance: Extra whitish band, usually bordering a lacuna

Meaning: Increased irritation or inflammation in the local area.

Physical Integrity #11 - Pinguecula

Appearance: Deposit of yellowish fatty tissue on the sclera, usually at the midline 3 and 9 o'clock.

Meaning: Indicates either tissue response to sun, wind, sand, or glare, or indicator for disturbed fat metabolism and liver stress.

Physical Integrity #12 - Pterygium

Appearance: Thickened conjunctival tissue extending over the nasal cornea.

Meaning: Tissue that grows and can obscure underlying iris and interfere with vision if large enough. Usually occurs from the sun, wind, sand, glare, or as a stress reaction. Surgically removed, they re-grow approx—50% of the time.

Physical Integrity #13 - Rarefaction of Stoma

Appearance: Subtle or distinct tissue dropout in a limited area

Meaning: Decreased vitality or functional capacity in a specific area.

Physical Integrity #14 - Reflexive Signs

Appearance: Distinct singular or multiple white fibbers

Meaning: Indicate irritation and inflammation in the local region. If pink or red, more reactive.

PART TWO

Secrets Of A Healer - Magic of Iridology

Eye Of The Beholder- Your Personality

Stream- Kinesthetic Type

Emotional Constitution Meaning:

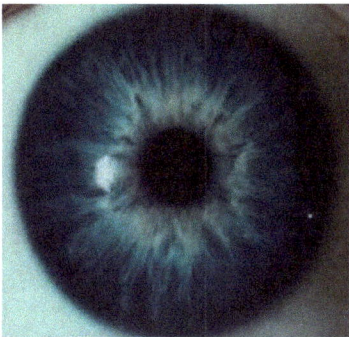

Stream Appearance: Neurogenic

Straight Lines (no flowers or flecks)

Quick Reference: Steady, Stable, Balancing, Support, Sensitive, Intuitive, Walking radar

Meaning:

Streams are subtle variations in the iris structure that appear as straight lines or wedges. Subtle variations in the fibers of the iris, which appear as straight lines or streaks of color, indicate a kinesthetic-type (stream) personality.

These physically oriented people tend to be intuitive yet consistently stable. Communicating and sensing with their bodies, they nurture and balance others. With genuine empathy, they mediate and integrate the extremes in society.

Periodically, their sensitivity becomes excessive, and they feel helplessly overwhelmed. Endowed with abundant physical energy and social skills, they are natural in healing and public service. However, their sense of being connected with people can lead to confusion about their self-worth or life purpose. By accepting the perfection in life and themselves, the kinesthetic type learns to touch others effectively without taking on unnecessary burdens. Stream-type structures indicate kinesthetic sensitivity, which learns best through experience.

They are attracted to people whose structures contain Jewel and Flower patterns (shakers).

Flower- Emotional Type

Emotional Constitution Meaning:

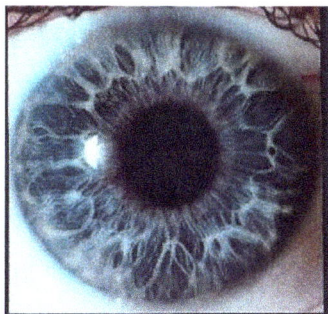

Appearance: Connective Tissue Flower Petals / Lacunas / Distinctly curved or rounded openings (flowers) in the fibers in the iris indicate an emotional-type person

Quick Reference: Seasonal, Transient, Brief but brilliant, Blossoming, Spontaneous, Changes a lot, Demonstrative, Social, on Stage.

Meaning:

These feeling-oriented people tend to be spontaneous, active, and changeable. Excellent visual communicator, animated and expressive, enjoy being on stage and flow easily with social situations. However, their passion for experiencing life and the tendency to over-commit can exhaust their energies, resulting in occasional bouts of depression or bursts of anger. Nevertheless, bubbling with enthusiasm and creative ideas, they make excellent engineers, artists, and musicians.

Quick to embrace new concepts, they add vitality to a project but often fail to see it through to completion. Learning to trust themselves, accept responsibility, and focus their energies enables emotional-type personalities to fulfill their desires successfully. Flower structures indicate an emotional disposition that learns best through auditory stimuli. They are attracted to Jewel-type individuals for long-term relationships.

Jewel- Mental Type

Emotional Constitution Meaning:

Appearance: Flecks / Jewels are dot-Like concentrations of color that can appear throughout the iris and range in color from light gold to black.

Quick Reference: Analytical, Thinking, Intellectual, Rational, Unemotional, Enduring, Slow to change, Increased self-control.

Meaning: Dot-like pigments (jewels) in the iris indicate a thinking intellectually oriented person. Mental-type personalities direct their active feelings through internal thought and analysis. Precise verbal communicators tend to control themselves, situations, and other people.

They generally show little emotion, and their gestures are few and pointed. Often intense, quietly frustrated people, their attention to detail can prove stifling to realizing their highest potential. Yet, having well-defined views, they often excel as teachers, leaders, and scientists.

These self-oriented individuals are slow to accept new ideas, yet having thoroughly analyzed the possibilities, they often lead the way. Learning to flow with situations and trust people enables mental-type personalities to better express their feelings and attain long-term goals. The disposition which learns best through visual stimuli. They are attracted to Flower-type individuals for long-term relationships.

Shaker- Extremist Type

Emotional Constitution Meaning:

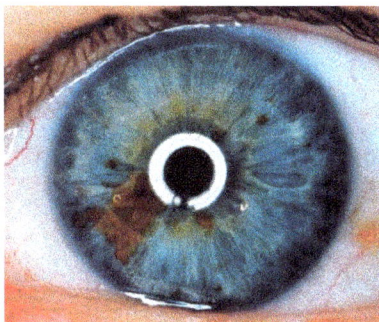

Appearance: Both, Flecks / Jewel <u>and</u> Lacunas/ Flowers/petals

The iris's dot-like pigments and distinct openings indicate an extremist-type (shaker) personality.

Quick Reference: Lacks moderation, Mover, Shaker, Accomplishments, Breaks the mold, Pioneers, Intense, Extremes in success and failures,

Meaning:

These action-oriented people tend to be dynamic and progressive individuals. Unifying visual and verbal modes of communication, their radical nature propels them to the forefront of change and innovation in society. However, because of their compelling drive and inherent instability, they experience incredible success and failure patterns, often exhausting their physical strength.

Characteristically devoted to a cause, they make excellent inventors, explorers, and motivators. Acting as the conscience of society, they often stand alone, attracting ridicule from their peers. Learning moderation and consistency enables the extremist-type personality to manifest change with stability.

Emotional Constitution Subtypes:

Ring of Freedom / Achievement rings

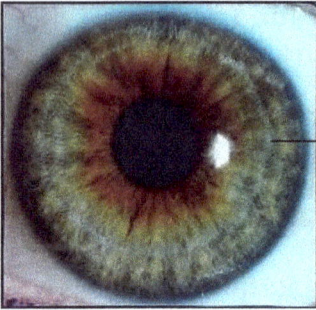

Appearance: Contraction furrows

Meaning: This person is a go, go, go, person. A doer, always busy, cannot relax and sit still.

Greatest strength: Motivation to produce.

Ring of Harmony

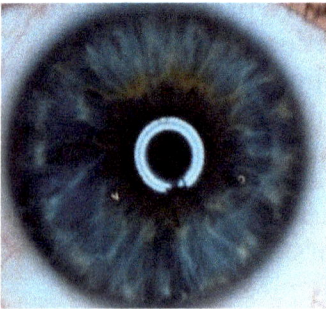

Appearance: Hydrogenoid / Uric Acid (Cotton balls)

Meaning: This person tries to make everyone happy.

Greatest strength: Influencing others

Tophi (tiny cotton balls) connective tissue bundles - in the outer ciliary 3 zone. It can range in appearance from distinct to poorly defined and from white to discolored.

Ring of Determination

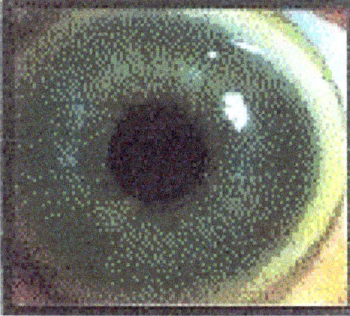

Appearance: Corneal Arcus / Cholesterol Ring / Lipemic Diathesis

Meaning: This person will not take no for an answer, they will prove anyone wrong, and they will always go the extra mile.

Greatest strength: Determination and boldness.

Ring of Purpose

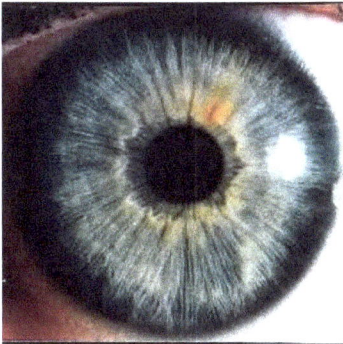

Appearance: Darker ring / Scruf ring *Darker distinct ring in outer ciliary 3 zone*

Meaning: This person will know what he/she is doing in life, Capable of anything, and may seem arrogant or confident.

Greatest strength: poise, calmness

Direction of Energy Flow:

Inward (Introvert)

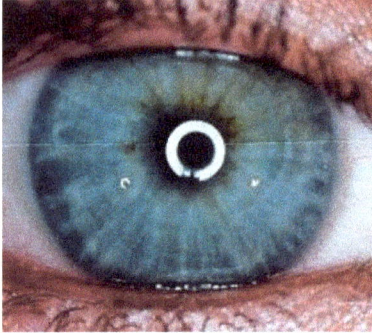

The energy of the anatomic nerve ring (digestive zone ring) is going toward the pupil.

• Sensitive, tolerant, insightful, quiet and observant, stability, empathy, integration, appreciation

Outward (Extrovert)

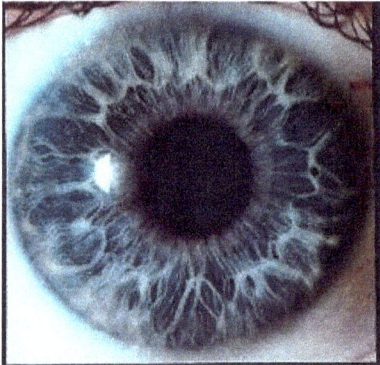

The energy of the anatomic nerve ring is going away from the pupil.

• Social, practical, expressive, honest, and directness, good at manifesting, coordination

Note: One of the best emotional/physical books to buy is: "Heal Your Body" by Louise L. Hay
ISBN; 9-780937-611357

Brain Hemisphere Dominance

If there are more markings, bigger markings, or more colors in one eye than the other, you will consider that eye with more markings the dominant eye.

You can also check by:

- What side of the bed do you sleep on?
- Which thumb is on top when they interlace your fingers?
- Which leg do you cross over the other?

People can also be balanced.

Left brain (analytical) Meaning

The majority of markings are in the RIGHT eye

- Fixed, doubtful, traditional, slow to change, logical, practical, compulsively ordered, restless, materialistic, questioning, contradictory, and fearful of being alone.

Right brain (creative)

The majority of markings are in the LEFT eye

- Spontaneous, accepting, future-oriented, creative, imaginative, intuitive, easygoing, sociable, and fear of rejection.

Note: Also, depending on which eye has markings, it is known that the left side is feminine, and the right is masculine. *Meaning; the markings in the right eye may mean you have more issues with men and vice–versa, women.*

Fun Facts

One of the most interesting books you might read is by;

Denny Ray Johnson book, "What the Eye Reveals" ISBN 0-91-7197-04-6

He has for each lacuna or fleck placement in the iris emotional meaning.

The one I have tested for years with my clients is the 3:00 o'clock and 9:00 o'clock marking.

Right   Left

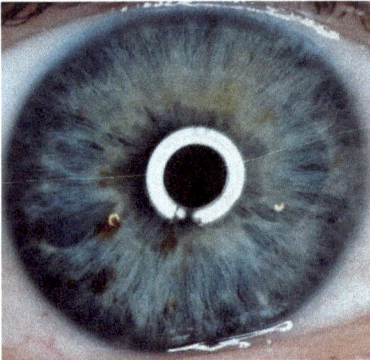 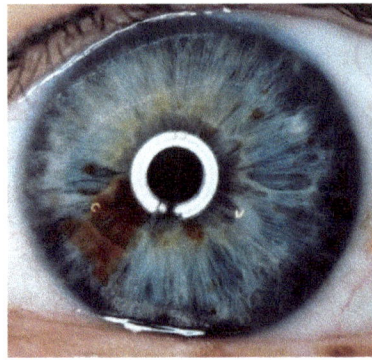

Notice the lacunas at 9:00 o'clock in her right eye and 3:00 o'clock in her left eye. When there are markings (lacunas or flecks) in these two locations, the parents are divorced 99% of the time. If not, they probably should be.

You can also tell who caused the issues or fighting; by the more prominent or more marks in that area. The left eye is Mom, and the right eye is Dad. The same is accurate for who you get along with more, mom or dad. Fewer markings that are who you get along better with. More markings, which you don't get along with.

Emotional Constitution

(Rayid Evaluation)

1) Pupil & Digestive Zone dominance?

> **Right Eye**   **Left Eye** _____

> _____

2) **Emotional Constitution**

Stream (straight lines) *steady*

_____   _____

Flower (lacunas) *emotional*

_____   _____

Jewel (flecks)   *analytical*

_____   _____

Shaker (fleck/lacunas) *mover*

_____   _____

3) Brain **Hemisphere Dominance**

Eye	Thumb	Legs	Bed
Right eye_____	R_____	R_____	R_____

= _____ Left-brained/*analytical*

| Left eye _____ | L_____ | L_____ | L_____ |

= _____ Right-brained/*creative*

4) Direction of Flow

Right eye / male Left eye/female

Balanced	_____	_____
Inward/*introvert*	_____	_____
Outwards/*extrovert*	_____	_____

5) Subtypes (Scale 1-10)

Ring of <u>freedom</u> (contraction)

1 2 3 4 5 6 7 8 9 10   1 2 3 4 5 6 7 8 9 10

None __   None __

Ring of <u>harmony</u> (hydrogeniod/uric acid)

1 2 3 4 5 6 7 8 9 10   1 2 3 4 5 6 7 8 9 10

None __   None __

Ring of <u>purpose</u> (scurf rim)

1 2 3 4 5 6 7   1 2 3 4 5 6 7

None __   None __

Ring of <u>determination</u> (lipemic)

1 2 3 4 5 6 7 8 9 10 1 2 3 4 5 6 7 8 9 10

None __   None __

Now What?

STAY HEALTHY!
A positive attitude is beneficial in healing, and the appropriate modality will benefit all body systems, reduce stress, improve circulation, and bring the body back to homeostasis.

Some suggestions for healing

Aromatherapy, Bach Remedy, Homeopathy

Emotional Clearing Technique

Energy Work, such as Reiki

Herbs, Vitamins & Supplements

Hypnosis, NLP, Inner Genie Work, or Meditation

Massage: such as ELD, Hot Stone, Swedish, Chair

Muscle Testing (Kinesiology), Body Talk

Quantum Medicine

Reflexology - Foot or Hand, Table Shiatsu, Acupressure or Acupuncture

Start Charting

PUTTING IT ALL TOGETHER

When clients come in, I love looking into their eyes and comparing my findings to their complaints. Iridology gives me a tool to chart a pattern to the client's issues. Iridology tells me what they were born with, Reflexology relates to me what they have been doing to their body since they got here, massage tells me where they hold their stress in their body, and muscle testing tells me anything I can get a yes/no answer to.

It's time to have fun looking at your own eyes and then looking at someone's eyes. Then, start to evaluate by getting an idea of your overall resiliency.

Following is a simplified version of an Iridology Chart I use for my clients

Check both eyes quickly, write down first thing you noticed.

Right eye _____   Left eye _____

Physical Integrity					Scale (1 is bad 10 is good)						Balanced

Resiliency	R	1	2	3	4	5	6	7	8	9	10
	L	1	2	3	4	5	6	7	8	9	10

Resiliency Subtypes		Connective Tissue				Polyglandular			Neurogenic		
	R	1	2	3	4	5	6	7	8	9	10
	L	1	2	3	4	5	6	7	8	9	10

Resiliency Modifiers

Contraction Furrows	R	1	2	3	4	5	6	7	8	9	10
	L	1	2	3	4	5	6	7	8	9	10

Digestive Zone

Placement	R	1	2	3	4	5	6	7	8	9	10
	L	1	2	3	4	5	6	7	8	9	10
Quality	R	1	2	3	4	5	6	7	8	9	10
	L	1	2	3	4	5	6	7	8	9	10
Shape	R	1	2	3	4	5	6	7	8	9	10
	L	1	2	3	4	5	6	7	8	9	10

Iris Constitution

	Lymphatic				Mixed Biliary			Hematogenic			
Over Acid	1	2	3	4							
Febrile		1	2	3	4						
Hydrogenoid	1	2	3	4	5	6	7	Tophi Color _____			
Uric Acid	1	2	3	4				Tophi Color _____			
Scurf Rim	1	2	3	4	5	6	7				
Ferrum Chromatose				4	5	6	7				
Lipemic Diathesis	1	2	3	4	5	6	7	8	9	10	
Over all Resiliency	1	2	3	4	5	6	7	8	9	10	

(Neurogenic increases over all resiliency)

Get a blank piece of paper ready to make notes.

1st Physical Integrity
Your Overall Resiliency Total # is _____

2nd Write down one point for each Iridology structural marking (Placement of lacunas and flecks, pigment colors, and any miscellaneous iris modifiers) you find in your eyes.

After adding all the checkmarks in each system, you will place the total on the systems chart.

Any system that has three or more marks needs to be looked after. The higher the marks, the higher the chances of issues and stress on that system.

3rd, Have fun doing your Emotional Integrity

Mock Charting - Physical

Iridology Case Study

Use this diagram to note all the markings you find (looking at a person).

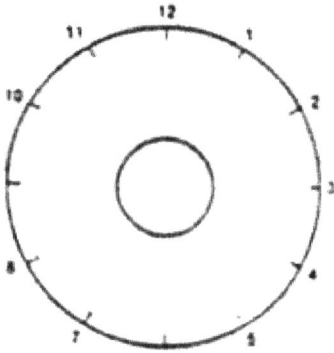

Their Right Eye   Their Left Eye

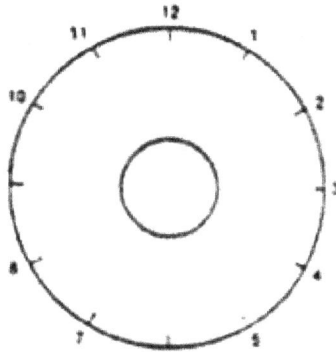

If you were doing an actual client's chart, you would legally have to use a black or blue pen to write with. Written with a pencil is not legal or professional.

1st) Have you ever had an eye injury?

Yes ___ No ___   _____

Have you ever had an eye surgery or laser treatment?

Yes ___ No ___ _____

Do you wear contact lenses?

Yes ___ No ___ Color _____

2nd) Check both eyes quickly. Write down the first thing you noticed.

Right eye _____ Left eye _____

3rd)

<u>**Physical Integrity**</u> I - V

Scale (1 is bad & 10 is good)

Balanced

I- Resiliency (your first instincts)

R   1 2 3 4 5 6 7 8 9 10

L   1 2 3 4 5 6 7 8 9 10

II- Resiliency Subtypes

	Connective Tissue	Polyglandular	Neurogenic
R	1 2 3 4	5 6 7	8 9 10
L	1 2 3 4	5 6 7	8 9 10

III- Resiliency Modifiers

A- Contraction Furrows

Lots & deep   Hardly any and faint

R	1	2	3	4	5	6	7	8	9	10
L	1	2	3	4	5	6	7	8	9	10

B- Digestive Zone

Placement

R	1	2	3	4	5	6	7	8	9	10
L	1	2	3	4	5	6	7	8	9	10

Quality

R	1	2	3	4	5	6	7	8	9	10
L	1	2	3	4	5	6	7	8	9	10

Shape

R	1	2	3	4	5	6	7	8	9	10
L	1	2	3	4	5	6	7	8	9	10

IV- Iris Constitution

Lymphatic   Mixed Biliary Hematogenic

Over Acid or Febrile   (Blue eyes only)

1 2 3 4

Hydrogenoid or Uric Acid   Tophi Color _____

1 2 3 4   5 6

Scurf Rim

1 2 3 4   5 6 7

Ferrum Chromatose   (Brown eyes only)

5 6 7 8

Lipemic Diathesis

1   2   3   4   5   6   7   8   9   10

V- Overall Resiliency

1   2   3   4   5   6   7   8   9   10

(Add up all circled numbers and divide by the number of circles you circled)

Ten is perfect and exceptionally resilient. They bounce back very fast!

E) Structural Signs (markings)

One checkmark in the system for <u>each</u> structural sign for;

Lacuna, rarefactions, transversals, topostable/topolabile flecks, sectoral heterochromia, defects

If there is a colored fleck, Check mark in the system also

		Left Eye	Right Eye
Allergies	Lymphatic		
	Over acid / Febrile		
Circulatory			
	Pupil		
	Hematogenic		
	Lipemic Diathesis		
	Neurogenic		
	Uric Acid		
	Heart		
Digestive			
	Orange		
	Fluorescent orange		
	Brown		
	Black		
	Polyglandular		
	Central Heterochromia		
	Connective		
	Lymphatic		
	Mixed / Biliary		
	Hematogenic		

	Throat / Esophagus		
	Gall Bladder		
	Liver		
	Ferrum Chromatose		
	Large Intestine/Colon		
	Pancreas		
	Rectum/Anus		
	Small Intestine/Colon		
	Stomach		
	Placement		
	Quality		
	Shape		
	Pupil		
Endocrine			
	Pupil		
	Polyglandular		
	Hematogenic		
	Adrenal		
	Pituitary		
	Pineal		
	Hypothalamus		
	Thyroid		
	Thymus		
	Pancreas		
	Ovaries/Testies		
Headache			
	Pupil		
	Neurogenic		
Immune			
	Hygrogenoid		
	Lymphatic		

	Mucus		
	Scurf Rim		
	Appendix		
	Sinus		
	Spleen		
	Tonsils		
Integument			
	Scurf Rim		
	Skin		
Lymphatic			
	Lymph		
	Hygrogenoid		
Muscular			
	Pupil		
	Muscles		
	Radial Furrows		
	Radial Solaris/ Parasites		
Neurological			
	Pupil		
	Autonomic Nervous		
	Brain		
	Medulla		
	Solar Plexus		
Reproductive			
	Pupil		
	Breast		
	Ovaries/Testis		
	Uterus/Prostate		
Respiratory			
	Pupil		
	Trachea		
	Diaphragm		
	Lung		
Senses			

	Pupil		
	Eyes (Sight)		
	Ears (Hearing)		
	Mouth (Taste)		
	Nose (Smell)		
	Sinus		
	Skin (Touch)		
Skeletal			
	Arthritic Netting		
	Pupil		
	Connective		
	Back Upper		
	Back Middle		
	Back Lower		
Urinary			
	Pupil		
	Uric Acid		
	Straw yellow		
	Bladder		
	Kidney		
Tumor /cancerous			
	Black flecks		
	Transferals		
	Pupil		

F) Emotional Constitution (Rayid Evaluation)

Constitution	Left Eye	Right Eye
Stream (straight lines) *steady*		
Flower (lacunas) *emotional*		
Jewel (flecks) *analytical*		
Shaker (fleck/lacunas) *mover*		

Brain Hemisphere Dominance

	Eye	Thumb	Legs	Bed
Right eye				
Left eye				

       More on Right   = Left-brained/analytical

       More on Left   = Right-brained/creative

Direction of Flow	Left Eye	Right Eye
	Female __	Male __
Balanced		
Inward / *introvert*		
Outward / *extrovert*		

Subtypes (Transfer from physical integrity page)

Ring of freedom (contraction)

      Left Eye   Right Eye

      1 2 3 4 5 6 7 8 9 10   1 2 3 4 5 6 7 8 9 10

Ring of harmony (hydrogeniod/uric acid)

      1 2 3 4 5 6 7 8 9 10   1 2 3 4 5 6 7 8 9 10

Ring of purpose (scurf rim)

      1 2 3 4 5 6 7   1 2 3 4 5 6 7

Ring of determination (lipemic)

      1 2 3 4 5 6 7 8 9 10   1 2 3 4 5 6 7 8 9 10

Quick Reference on Client Chart

Section A

There are a few questions to have the client answer.

Section B

This sometimes matters because your intuition seems to sense something important.

Section C

This will tell you individual information plus the overall resiliency of the client's constitution (how fast they bounce back from an illness).

Section D

Pupil information can count towards the system chart.

Section E

Systems of the body are shown in the eye.

Look for the mark first, starting at <u>one o'clock</u> in the person's eye and then proceeding around the clock and then to the other eye. (look at the person's eye for a mark, then transfer to the form).

If there is something you would like to add, write it in the corresponding system.

You may have more than one mark in any system.

There also will be many systems with no marks.

One checkmark for each (fleck, lacuna, rarefaction, color, etc.) in each eye for all systems system that has something. Some systems will have nothing at all.

Section F

This will give you emotional/personality information about the client.

With the info from sections C-E (add up all the marks), you will use this chart type to show the number of marks in each system.

Hypothetical Example:

Systems Chart

	Health Chart	Iridology
Skeletal	11	
Muscular		1111
Nervous		
Circulatory	1	
Urinary		
Reproductive	1	
Digestive		
Endocrine	111	1
Immune		
Lymphatic		
Respiratory		
Senses		

*From your findings, you will notice that the client's Muscle and Endocrine systems both have four marks. These are the two systems to share with clients to ensure they keep healthy, preventative medicine.

Transfer info: # of marks

Systems Chart	Health Chart	Iridology	Reflex	Muscle Testing	Massage
Skeletal					
Muscular					
Nervous					
Circulatory					
Urinary					
Reproductive					
Digestive					
Endocrine					
Immune					
Lymphatic					
Respiratory					
Senses					

Iridology Homework

Have Fun!

1) Who originally discovered Iridology?

   _____

2) How did he discover Iridology? What happened?

   _____
   _____
   _____
   _____

3) Who wrote the book 'Diagnosis from the Eye'?

   _____

4) Match the description with the parts of the eye:

Pupil	_____	A) Is the white of the eye, often containing visible blood vessels.
Cornea	_____	B) The transparent layer of tissue covers the eyeball.
Lens	_____	C) A colored, muscular ring that controls the amount of light entering the eye.
Iris	_____	D) Which allows the focusing of light on the back of the inside of the eyeball.
Sclera	_____	E) Is the aperture within the iris which allows light to enter the eye.

5)   How many markings does it take even to mean there may be a severe issue/trait?

_____

6)   What tool do you need to read the eyes with?

_____

7)   Give a brief description of the two belief systems?

_____
_____
_____

8)   What are the three principles in Hering's Law of Cure?

_____
_____
_____
_____
_____
_____

9)   Describe what a healing crisis is?

_____
_____
_____
_____
_____
_____

10) In the boxes, fill in the eye color of the children.

      A)   <u>Parent A</u>

                   b   b
<u>Parent B</u>
      B
      b

B)

Parent A

	B	B
Parent B		
B		
B		

11) What is the eye color % from questions 10-A?

_____

12) What is the eye color % from questions 10-B?

_____

13) Describe a lacuna?

_____
_____

14) Describe the appearance of a lacuna?

_____
_____

15) What color can the iris pigmentation flecks be?

What organ(s) does it relate to?

_____   _____
_____   _____
_____   _____
_____   _____
_____   _____

16)Describe what a radial furrow would appear like in the eye?

_____

_____

17) Describe what the scurf rim would appear like in the eye?

_____

_____

18) Describe what ferrum chromatose would appear like in the eye?

_____

_____

19) Describe what topolabile pigments would appear like in the eye?

_____

_____

20) What determines the Iris Resiliency/Constitution?

_____

_____

21) What are the three physical resiliency subtypes?

_____

_____

_____

22) What do contraction furrows indicate?

_____

_____

23) What is the digestive wreath also known as?

_____

_____

24) What are the three iris constitutions or genotypes?
Answer:

_____

_____

_____

25) Describe what over acid would appear like in the eye?

_____

_____

Iridology Homework Answer Key

1)Who originally discovered Iridology?
Answer:
 Dr. Ignatz von Peczely

2)How did he discover Iridology? What happened?
Answer:
A boy was playing with an owl & the owl's leg broke. The boy noticed a line that formed in the owl's eye.

3)Who wrote the book "Diagnosis from the Eye?"
Answer:
Nils Liljequist.

4)Match the description with the parts of the eye:
A) Pupil   Answer: E
B) Cornea   Answer: B
C) Lens   Answer: D
D) Iris   Answer: C
E) Sclera   Answer: A

5) How many markings does it take even to mean there may be a severe issue/trait?
 Answer:
4 - 5

6) What tool do you need to read the eyes with?
Answer:
Lighted magnified glass

7) Give a brief description of the two belief systems?
Answer:
(1)   The iris markings Do Not change over a person's life.
(2)   The iris markings Can Change & is just a snapshot

of the eye at that moment.

8) What are the three principles in Hering's Law of Cure?
Answer:
A) All cure comes from above downward.
B) All cure comes from within out.
C) All symptoms leave the body in the reverse order they entered.

9) Describe what a healing crisis is?
Answer:
A healing crisis is when the body has gained enough vital energy to eliminate some of the accumulated toxins in the devitalized tissue.

10) In the boxes, fill in the eye color of the children.
Answer:
A)

Bb	Bb
bb	bb

B)

BB	BB
BB	BB

11) What is the eye color % from questions 10-A?
Answer:
hybrid 50% & blue 50%

12) What is the eye color % from questions 10-B?
Answer:
100% true brown.

13) Describe a Lacuna?
Answer:
Pit, hole, relating to lacune or lake, flower

14) Describe the appearance of a lacuna?
Answer:
Distinctly rounded deficiency of tissue. It resembles a flower petal.

15) What color can the iris pigmentation flecks be? What organ(s) does it relate to?
Answer:

Color	Meaning
Straw Yellow -	Kidney
Orange -	Pancreas and Liver
Fluorescent Orange -	Gallbladder, Pancreas, Liver
Brown	Liver
Black/Tar -	Pre-cancerous and Liver

16)Describe what a radial furrow would appear like in the eye?
Answer:
This indicates increased toxic material in the adjacent and surrounding tissue.

17) Describe what the scurf rim would appear like in the eye?
Answer:
Darker distinct ring on the outer ciliary zone.

18) Describe what ferrum chromatose would appear like in the eye?

Answer:
Tiger stripes are bands of small dark "snuff tobacco" pigments that accumulate on the surface of the iris.

19) Describe what topolabile pigments would appear like in the eye?
Answer:
Flecks, general pigment pattern scattered through the iris.

20) What determines the Iris Resiliency/Constitution?
Answer:
The closer the fibers are, the more resiliency.

21) What are the three physical resiliency subtypes?
Answer:
a) Neurogenic
b) Connective tissue
c) Polyglandular

22) What do contraction furrows indicate?
Answer:
Attraction to stress.

23) What is the digestive wreath also known as?
Answer:
Bowel wreath or autonomic nerve wreath.

24) What are the three iris constitutions or genotypes?
Answer:
a) Lymphatic
b) Mixed biliary
c) Hematogenic

25) Describe what over acid would appear like in the eye?
Answer:
Blue eye with whitish fibers.

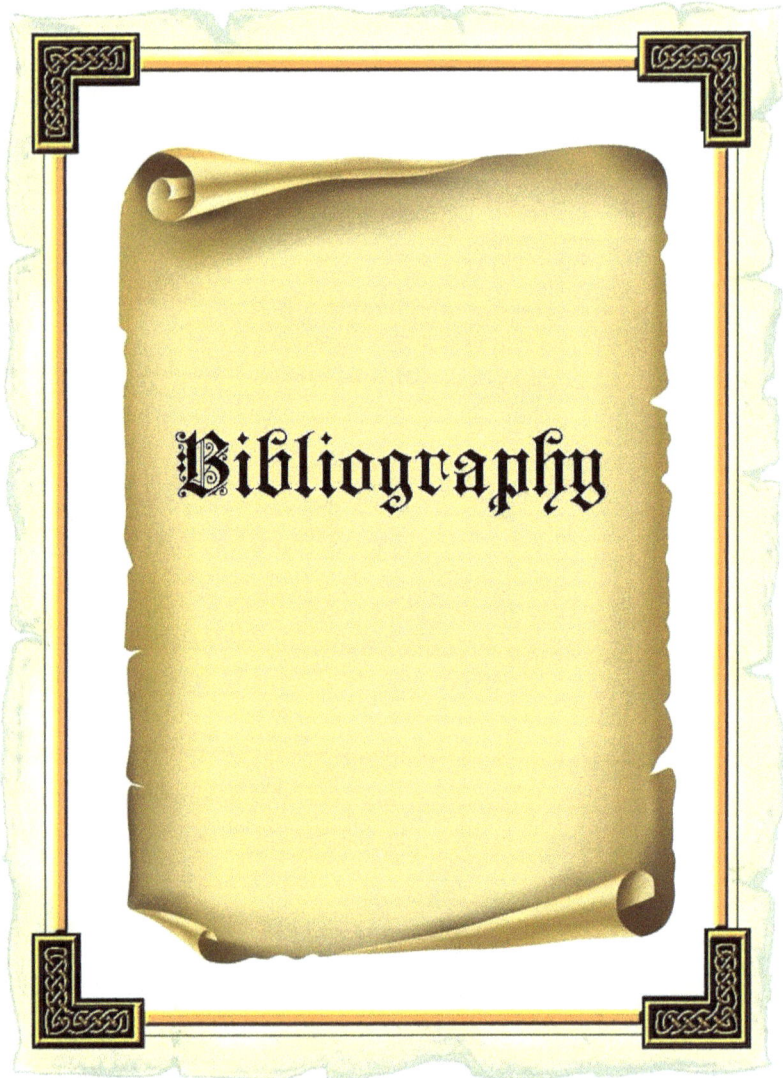

Bibliography

Bibliography

Much of this information was taken from the course information created when I owned the Canadian Institute Of Natural Health And Healing Accredited College.

Physical Integrity

Caradonna, Bill Dr. Applied Iridology. 1998

Jensen, Bernard, D.C., Ph.D. Iridology The Science and Practice in the Healing Arts Vol II 1982

Tart-Jensen, Ellen. Techniques in Iris Analysis Part 1. Video series

Bamer, Dr. Donald R. Practical Iridology, and Sclerology. ISBN 1-885670-02-8

Magda, D. Carol. Iridology A focused Study. 2004

Emotional Integrity

Johnson, Denny Ray. What the Eye Reveals. 1995

Micaller, ElizabethPh.D. Emotional Iridology and the Body Mind Connection.

A Grand Medicine Manual, Personality Iridology Iris 2. 2005

Charts

My Chart was created and copyrighted using a blend of Dr Bernard Jensen, Dr. Bill Caradonna, and Dr. Peczely's Charts

Message From The Author

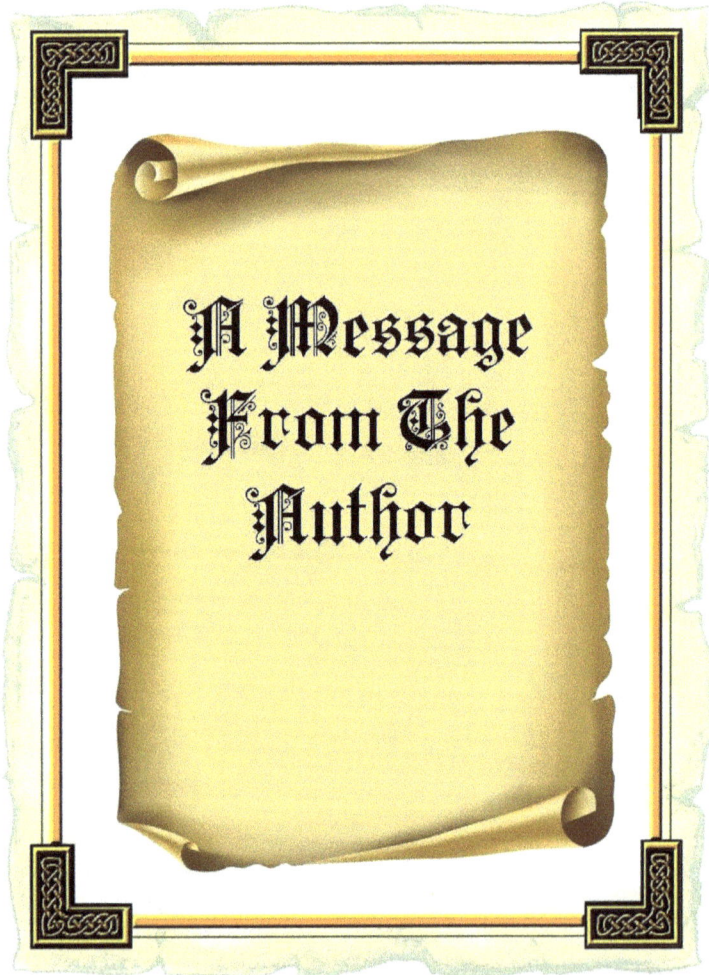

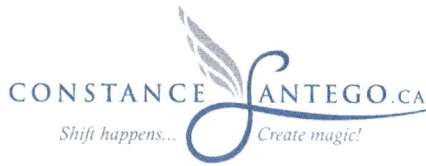

Too bad I don't have pictures to see the details of my eyes at age one. I would love to know if I have always had different colored eyes or just after the accident.

I had an accident and was blinded in my left eye at the age of one and a half. At eleven, due to a cataract forming, I needed an operation to remove my lens.

The first time I went to have my eyes looked at by an Iridologist was in 1992. The pictures of my eyes were taken with a different camera each year, so the color changes are not actual year to year.

As you can see in my left eye, I have a black mark at about 1:00 o'clock; it is not cancer. When the doctor removed my last stitch, some tissue came away with it. You will also notice my pupil is egg-shaped; this is not a tumor. Back in the day, there was no laser treatment. The doctor had to cut around my iris, remove the lens, and sew me back up. The odd shape is due to having no lens and the tissue being damaged.

What you should be able to tell about me;

- I have a scruff rim; I need a purpose in my life.
- Contraction furrows; I'm a go, go, go, person
- Digestive issues
- I have markings in both 3 and 9 o'clock; divorced parents

My Right   My Left

1992

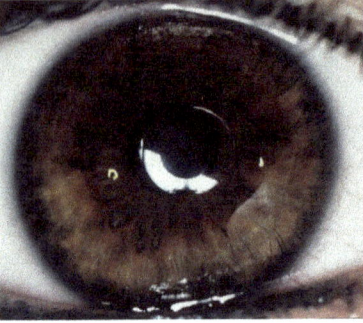 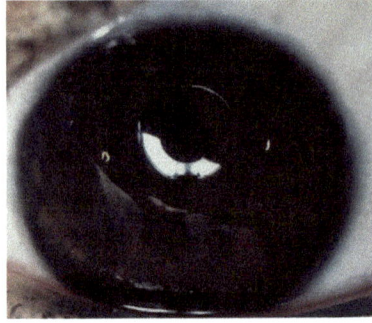

2003

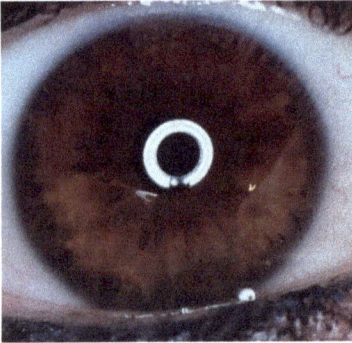 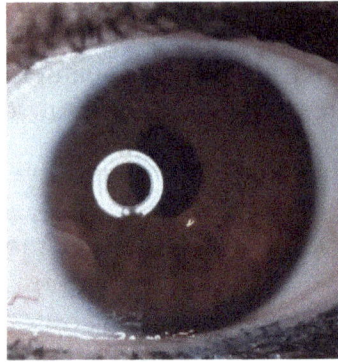

2011

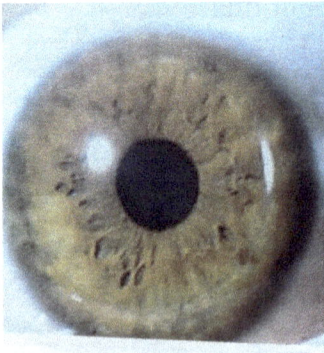 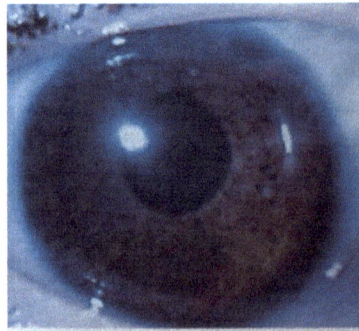

Dec 2019

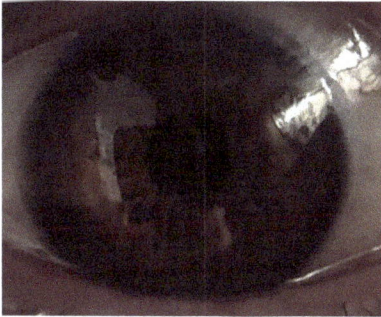

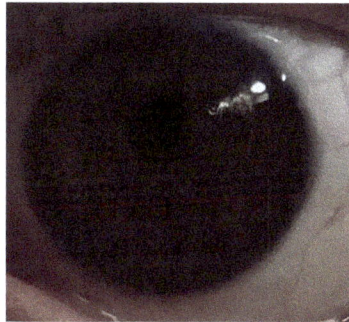

P.S. Iridology is a tool that I use to tell me what health my client was given at birth and what system(s) in the body are their main issues of concern.

I love the personality aspect; it is dead on every time.

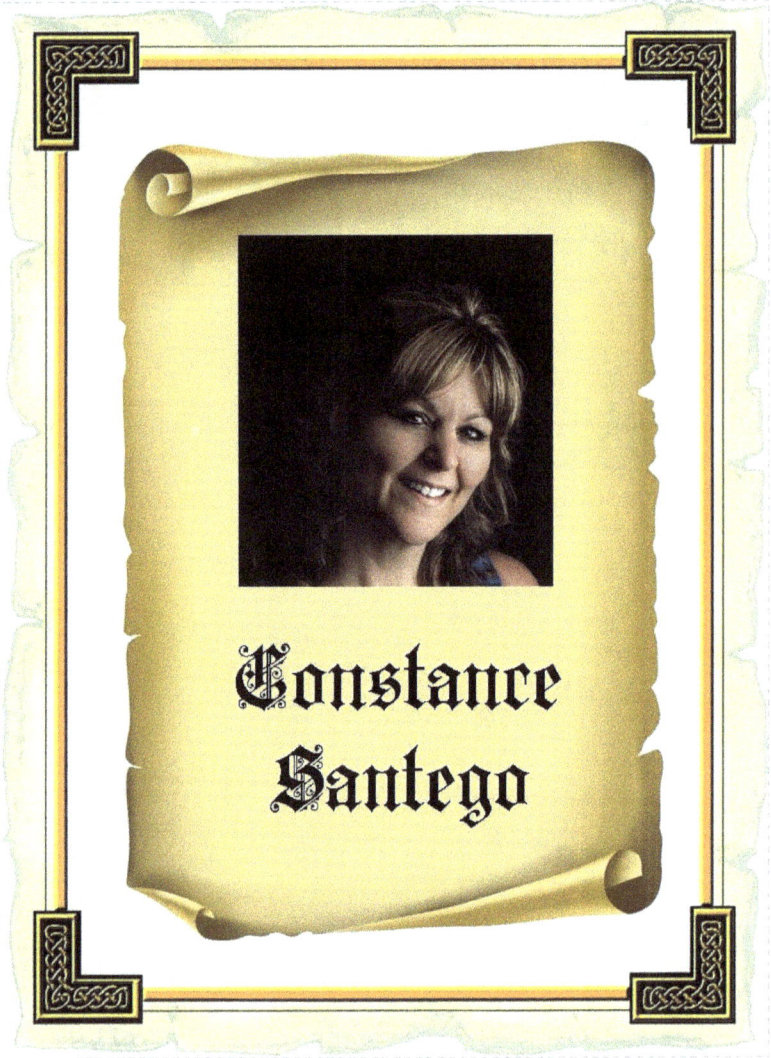

Shift happens...Create magic!
Dream BIGGER!

Dr. Constance Santego is a highly respected expert in the field of holistic health and spiritual healing. With over twenty years of experience teaching courses on these subjects, she has developed a deep understanding of the interconnectedness of the mind, body, and spirit in achieving overall well-being.

Dr. Santego holds a Ph.D. and Doctorate in Natural Medicine, which has provided her with a comprehensive understanding of alternative healing modalities and their application in promoting optimal health. Her educational background has equipped her with the knowledge to address health concerns from a holistic perspective, considering the physical, emotional, and spiritual aspects of an individual's well-being.

Throughout her career, Dr. Santego has been committed to sharing her knowledge and empowering others to take control of their health and healing. She has a unique ability to blend scientific research and traditional wisdom, creating a bridge between conventional and alternative medicine.

In her "Secrets of a Healer" educational series, Dr. Santego draws upon her vast experience and expertise to captivate readers with her insights and teachings. She takes readers on a transformative journey, delving into the realms of holistic health, spirituality, and self-discovery. Through her writing, she aims to inspire individuals to tap into their own innate healing abilities and embrace a balanced and harmonious approach to well-being.

Dr. Santego's work has touched the lives of many, guiding them toward a more profound understanding of themselves and their connection to the world around them. Her series serves as a beacon of wisdom, offering practical tools and techniques for personal growth and transformation.

Overall, Dr. Constance Santego's blend of knowledge, experience, and passion makes her a captivating figure in the field of holistic health and spiritual healing. Her contributions through teaching, writing, and her spellbinding series continue to inspire and empower individuals on their journeys toward well-being and self-discovery.

ALSO AVAILABLE

Play the game *Ikona* – Discover Your Inner Genie

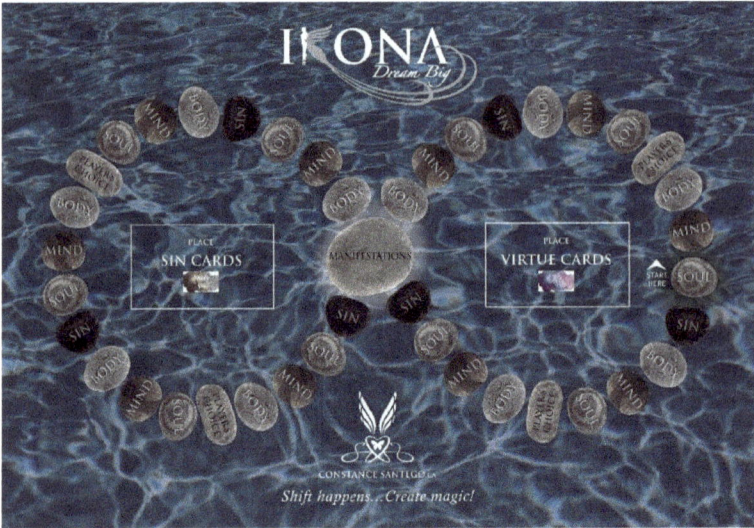

For additional information on

Constance Santego's

wide range of Motivational Products, Coaching Sessions,
Spiritual Retreats,
Live Events and Educational Programs

Go to

www.ConstanceSantego.ca

Follow on Instagram - Constance_Santego &
Facebook - constancesantegoo

Subscribe and receive free information and Meditations on my
YouTube Channel - Constance Santego

NOTES:

www.ingramcontent.com/pod-product-compliance
Lightning Source LLC
Chambersburg PA
CBHW072132020426
42334CB00018B/1771